Praise for the Third [illegible] of *Coming Home*

"Thank you for the joy you shared with our poor through your gift."

—Mother Teresa

"[An] exce[illegible]ne practical understanding about [illegible], as well as the resources available in this country. It is beautifully written, extremely helpful. I am proud of Deborah's work."

—Elisabeth Kübler-Ross, MD

"Highly recommended."

—*Library Journal*

"Teaches an important lesson to those of us who must confront the death of a loved one."

—*Los Angeles Times*

"A very important book that will be very useful."

—Jerry Jampolsky, MD

"A pioneering work. As a comprehensive resource book, it is invaluable for family and friends wishing to help an individual die at home."

—*Open Hands Quarterly*

"This is a book worth reading. In social transformation where financial resources alone may lead to more individuals to choosing to die at home, this is a worthwhile guide for lay persons and can be confidently recommended by health care professionals."

—C. Norman Shealy, MD, PhD

"Includes practical information that makes decisions about death and dying easier and kinder."

—Hugh Prather

Coming Home

A Practical and Compassionate Guide to Caring for a Dying Loved One

Deborah Duda

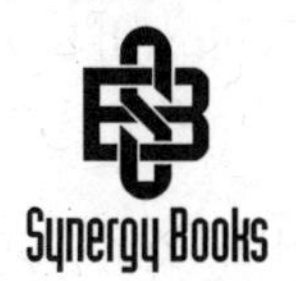

Coming Home: A Practical and Compassionate Guide to Caring for a Dying Loved One
Published by Synergy Books
P.O. Box 30071
Austin, Texas 78755

For more information about our books, please write us, e-mail us at info@synergybooks.net, or visit our web site at www.synergybooks.net.

Printed and bound in Canada.

The text of this book is printed on 100% post-consumer recycled paper.

Publisher's Cataloging-in-Publication
(Provided by Quality Books, Inc.)

Duda, Deborah.
Coming home : a practical and compassionate guide to caring for a dying loved one / Deborah Duda.
p. cm.
Includes bibliographical references.
LCCN 2010925622
ISBN-13: 978-0-9842358-9-6
ISBN-10: 0-9842358-9-2

1. Terminally ill--Home care. 2. Terminal care.
3. Death--Psychological aspects. 4. Caregivers.
5. Hospice care. I. Title.

R726.8.D856 2010 649.8
QBI10-600082

Author photo by Thomas Grollman, MD

10 9 8 7 6 5 4 3 2 1

To Eve Muir, my friend and family,
who made this book possible, and to
all the people who have had the love
and courage to care for their dying
loved ones at home.

TABLE OF CONTENTS

AUTHOR'S NOTE

The medical, health, and supportive procedures in this book are based on the training, personal experiences, and research of the author, and on recommendations of responsible medical and nursing sources. But because each person and situation is unique, the author and publisher urge the reader to check with a qualified health professional before using any procedure where there is any question as to its appropriateness.

Because some risks may be involved, the author and publisher assume no responsibility for any adverse effects or consequences resulting from the use of any of the suggestions, preparations, or procedures in this book. Please do not use the book if you are unwilling to assume those risks. Feel free to consult a physician or other qualified health professional. It is a sign of wisdom, not timidity or cowardice, to seek a second or third opinion.

PREFACE TO THE NEW EDITION

Coming Home was first published in 1981, followed by second and third editions in 1984 and 1987. The possibility of a new edition prompted me to review how far Americans have come in how we think about dying and how we care for people who are dying.

When I first became involved with death and dying in the late 1970s, there were two hospices in America: the Connecticut Hospice inspired by Dame Cicely Saunders, the English founder of the modern hospice movement, and the Hospice of Marin, in California. Dr. Elisabeth Kübler-Ross, whom I consider a mentor, was a crusader for humanizing how we as a society treated the dying. Her classic book *On Death and Dying* stood almost alone on the subject.

Now, in 2010, there are more than 4,850 hospices in America. Hospice care is within the reach of most Americans and has been covered by Medicare and Medicaid since 1982.

In those early days in the seventies, I'd never heard the phrase "palliative care," or its other name, "comfort care." The palliative care movement has grown out of the holistic health care movement and the hospice movement. It addresses symptoms, pain control, and the spiritual and psychosocial needs of patients and their families, extending the hospice concept of patient care to all people facing medical challenges. Palliative care is about making the practice of medicine kinder, and kindness is a joy wherever we find it. As the Dalai Lama said, "Kindness is my religion."

Now there are over five hundred palliative care units in U.S. hospitals. Young doctors study "comfort care" in medical school and carry its ideas and practices into whatever field of medicine they choose. I hope it won't be too long before there is a board-certified specialty in palliative care.

We've come a long way. Yet while most Americans say they would like to die at home, 50 percent die in hospitals. According to National Hospice and Palliative Care Organization statistics, only 38 percent of all U.S. deaths happened under a hospice program, and the remainder occurred in nursing homes.[1] The dying who enter a hospice program do so, on average, within the last ten days of their earthly lives.

If they entered a hospice program earlier and used all the hospice's skills for pain control, comfort, and emotional and spiritual support, they and their families might share a more healing, peaceful journey. But entering a hospice program is an acknowledgement that our loved one is dying, and we still find admitting that very difficult. Somewhat surprisingly, a study in the *Journal of Pain and Symptom Management* reported that hospice patients live, on average, twenty-nine days longer than non-hospice patients.[2]

In 2008, the American Association of Retired People (AARP) reported that 94 million Americans were in the fifty-plus age group.[3] A huge number of us will face dying sooner rather than later, and we'll have to make choices about what we want and what we don't want.

What is called end-of-life care is not only a personal issue, but also a pressing social, economic, and political issue for the United States. In 2008, 25 to 30 percent of Medicare expenditures were spent on care for patients' last year of earthly life. The price tag was one hundred billion dollars. How much of this was used for meaningful care to improve the quality of life, and how much was used to prolong the lives of people who might not have wanted the care if they had fully understood their choices? Clearly, unless we take more responsibility for dying, the final medical expenditures made on our behalf could bankrupt Medicare.

As I reviewed the earlier editions of *Coming Home,* I noticed that it had a scrappy crusader tone in many places that no longer seems necessary or appropriate. When I wrote the earlier editions, it seemed like I, and the many others concerned about quality of life, had to fight for the humane treatment of dying people. Therefore, in the new edition, I've not only updated all the information but also adjusted the book's tone to reflect my and society's maturing attitudes toward death and dying.

The earlier editions of *Coming Home* share stories of the deaths of two very close friends and my father. Since then, my mother had a quietly remarkable death, the memory of which consistently brings a smile to my face and heart. In considering all the work necessary to update and republish *Coming Home,* I decided that if I could help even a few families to have an uplifting memory of the death of someone they loved dearly, the work would be worthwhile.

So here we go! Bless you and your family on your journey. I imagine myself sitting at the kitchen table with you, cheering you on and learning with you.

Aloha,

Deborah Duda

In the Beginning there was Life. And Life seemed to be without form. It was indistinguishable. So Death was created to give form to Life. And then people began to become attached to Life and to see Death as the enemy. In some places people saw Life as the enemy, the place of suffering, and Death as the friend.

And now we come to a place where we see that both are One.

So those of us who made an enemy of Death must make of Death a friend. And those who made an enemy of Life must make of Life a friend.

INTRODUCTION

Some thirty years ago, I was wandering around the world, looking outside myself for some teacher or teaching to help me understand what my life was all about. I decided to return to the clarity I remembered feeling while hiking through a small village at the foot of Mount Machapuchare in Nepal.

In Pokhara, I found a Sherpa guide who volunteered to act as an interpreter and go with me to the village to find a house. The next day, two Tibetan women carried my bags up the mountain trails to the tiny mud house we had found, and I set up housekeeping. I quit trying to figure it all out and just lived contentedly with the villagers, taking photographs and recording the sounds and music of village life.

After a few weeks, I began to have nightmares that I or someone in my family was dying. Each day, I was afraid of what the next night might bring. One day a few months later, a Sherpa stopped by with a Valentine's Day card from my parents and a copy of *Newsweek* magazine with Mother Teresa's picture on the cover. That night, I dreamed about her.

The next morning, I decided the only way to overcome my fear of death was to put myself in the middle of it. I would go to Calcutta and ask Mother Teresa if I could work in a *hriday* house, one of the homes she created for people dying on the streets (*hriday* is Sanskrit for "heart").

By the time I arrived in Calcutta, I was so sick with dysentery and worms that getting out of bed to call Mother Teresa was a great effort. I dragged myself to a public telephone booth in a steamy Calcutta street, picked up the phone, and dialed the operator. I told the operator that I wanted to speak with Mother Teresa. In a few minutes, she was on the phone.

I found her easy to talk with. I told her about my dreams and asked if I could see her. Very lovingly, she said, "Come right over, my child."

I dragged myself to the main convent in Calcutta and asked her my crucial question: "Can I work for a few months in one of your homes for the dying?"

"No, my child," she said. "Go home. There is sadness and suffering right around you at home."

Then, feeling desperate and lonely, I asked, "Can I adopt a child from the orphanage?"

Again she answered, "No, my child. Go home and work with the sadness and loneliness around you."

And I did—first with the fear, sadness, and loneliness in myself. And the key has been *hriday*—the heart—and transforming the fear that keeps hearts closed.

I began writing the first edition of this book after two friends I loved very much were cared for at home until they died. Then I worked with terminally ill patients and their families at our local hospital, and with some who chose to die at home. While I was working on the final edit, my father died at home.

Before the deaths of my two friends, when I thought of dying, I felt stupid. That made me feel afraid or angry, so I feigned indifference. As a teenager, I had seen only one living thing die—a gray squirrel on a country road. I shuddered as I watched its death dance in the rearview mirror. Death on a public road! It was out of place—unnatural, even! Everyone knows animals go away to die in hidden places. For three days, I kept off the road, trying to figure out where this death fit into the scheme of things. Later in life, I shot a few deer, but I blanked that out. I saw my grandfather dead, but I didn't see how he got that way.

Not until I was past thirty did I really become aware that people were dying around me all the time, that *I* was dying all the time—parts of me, old cells, old ideas, old ways of being. Death was hidden in hospitals, in statistics, in a compartment of my being I didn't open. I saw a friend lonely and isolated because fear kept friends from talking with her about the most important thing happening in her life: her dying.

Then I was angry, truly angry. My anger was born from awareness of my own ignorance and fear. I felt cheated. Most of us are cheated out of the fullness of life by fear and embarrassment. We experience the pain and joy of birth and life, but many of us deny ourselves our deaths, the closure of a circle. Denial comes from fear: our fear, doctors' fear, loved ones' fear, our whole culture's fear.

As I began to accept dying and death as part of my life, my fear was transformed into love, my anger into compassion, my depression into joy. The quality of my relationships with myself and with others improved. Now, after working with dying people and experiencing the deaths and rebirths within myself, I feel more profoundly my kinship with all of life.

This book grew from a sense of our wholeness (holiness). It covers the practical information needed to help alleviate many of our fears. "Practical" includes not only the "what to do" and "how to do it" of physical care, but also mental, emotional, and spiritual support. Once the needs for comfort and relief from pain are met, spiritual food can be more nourishing than a glass of carrot juice or a hamburger. Supporting a home dying is an opportunity to learn that spiritual support can be practical, and physical care can be spiritual.

This book, then, is a synthesis of my psychological and spiritual understandings and the basic information on physical care needed to support someone who lives at home until he or she dies. It includes things to keep in mind when a loved one is deciding where to die, and, if home is the choice, what you can do about family morale, pacing yourself, pain relief, interacting with doctors, giving injections, taking care of your feelings, and so on. Although the book is directed principally to the family and friends of the dying person, much of it can be shared with the dying person as well.

I share with you my reality, my vision, at this time in my life. Your reality, including your spiritual understanding and approach to death, may be different. Use this book as a tool to help find the answers in yourself. If I use words that are not your words, let's move deeper than the word level to the level of the heart.

Trust yourself. We learn by having the courage to enter another's reality without seeing it as a threat, and we can do this only if we trust ourselves. Sometimes seeing ideas in print convinces us that someone out there is an expert who knows more than we do about our own experience. But anyone outside of ourselves can be only a provider of information or inspiration. You're the only expert on your reality. The appropriate way to support someone who is dying is the way the dying person and you choose. And if some of your choices are different from the dying person's, you can do it your way when it's your turn.

Dying is the process of the life forces withdrawing from the body, and death is the moment of withdrawal. We often hear that life and death are opposites. To me, the opposites are birth and death. One describes entering into form, the other leaving form—which is which depends on your perspective. Either way, life continues without end.

In this book, *dying, death,* and *died* refer only to a change in form and do not mean "the end," "the final disaster," "the worst thing that could happen," or "the uncontrollable enemy." I see death as a friend on our way home to more life, and caring for someone who is dying as an opportunity to serve as a midwife for a soul.

I believe that at some level of our being, we decide when we're going to die. After that, our only choices are our attitude about dying and, sometimes, where it will take place. Both affect the quality of the time we have, and the latter may affect the quantity.

Accepting death is a process of surrender, of letting go and accepting life as it *is* rather than as we think it *should* be. Exquisite beauty and meaning can be present in dying when we and the dying person accept in our hearts that life is following its natural course, and when we cooperate with life instead of fighting against it. When we do, we no longer feel separate from each other and from life; we experience the underlying unity of everything.

Love transforms fear. Caring for a dying person is an opportunity to increase our capacity to love by decreasing our fear. Within each of us is love, someone to love, and someone to love us. But fear keeps hearts closed, which prevents us from experiencing this. Fear prevents surrendering and makes us feel separate and alone.

Fear projects awful things that may happen, especially while someone is dying. I've never encountered anything awful in all the home dyings I've been involved with. Before I worked with dying people, I seemed to be the ideal candidate for not being able to handle dying. I had a long history of passing out in health class, at the sight of blood, or just when visiting a friend in the hospital. I was terrified each time I got a shot, and on more than one occasion, I threw up in reaction to someone near me vomiting.

But then I realized that to be afraid of death is to be afraid of life. This book is about acknowledging our fears and, at the same time, moving through them toward greater love, joy, and freedom as we experience dying.

One way our culture teaches fear of death is by making security a goal. Total security is, of course, an illusion. Life is a process of change, and inherent in change are vulnerability and risk. At any moment, our plans for the future can disintegrate. Holding on to security or chasing after it creates more insecurity and fear. And do we really want it anyway? Maximum security is prison, not life. We break the circle of fear and insecurity when we live each moment as it comes. You can live in the moment right now with this dying you're living.

Peace is possible in this moment. It's not out there somewhere in the future. The future never really comes, anyway; by the time it gets to us, it's the present.

Focusing on life as a process instead of a goal has helped me accept death. I accept that at any point in time, a process is complete up until that moment. At each moment, each of us is complete and whole. No one dies before the purpose of his or her life is fulfilled, even if we cannot understand that purpose. I believe that a child who dies young or someone who dies unexpectedly dies complete. Perhaps some of their projects aren't complete, but who we are is not our unfinished work, projects, or goals. The purpose of goals is just to give us a sense of direction.

When life is seen as a process and not as a goal, death loses much of its sting. As Chief Crazy Horse said, "Today is a good day to die, for all the things of my life are here."

Dying, like living, has its share of sadness and joy. The sadness of letting go of a person we love is tempered if we remember to hold everyone lightly, knowing they are "just on loan." When someone we love is dying, we tend to focus on sadness, not on joy. But it's a choice. We can allow joy into what is often the most painful experience of our lives: the quiet joy of sharing love and caring, of seeing a loved one content, of touching timelessness, of feeling connected with all of life.

If we live each moment of each day fully, we transcend time. Each moment then becomes an eternity, and we have all the time in the universe to share with this dying person we love. It doesn't matter how long we live, only *how* we live the time we have. It's possible to create from this experience a beautiful time in your life. And perhaps, if you allow joy into this experience, you will be surprised how often it erases emotional pain.

The increased love and compassion we can learn while caring for someone who dies at home help us through our initial loneliness. If the death has not been sudden, there's been time between smoothing sheets, emptying bedpans, holding hands, and talking of what may come for grieving and resolving anything we need to resolve with the dying person. There's been time to begin a gradual adjustment to earthly life without this person.

Because dying is living intensified, the qualities most needed to support someone who is dying are the same ones needed for living fully: love, compassion, courage, serenity, patience, humor, humility, and the will to let others live or die as they choose, as long as they take responsibility for their choices. I know you have some of those qualities, maybe all of them, and maybe even in great abundance.

By taking responsibility for dying, we reclaim responsibility for living and regain the personal power we've given away. One way to take responsibility is to stop playing victim to cultural pressure to go away quietly and die in the sterility of a nursing home or hospital. Who wants to be seen as a forthcoming vacancy? We can die right here amidst the people and things we love: the kids, the dog, the garden, our favorite chair.

As you live this dying, be gentle with yourself and love yourself. There's no need to judge yourself, blame yourself, or feel guilty. Our lives are a learning process in which we outgrow some old thoughts and feelings as we increase in wisdom. Guilt about the past is a way of punishing ourselves for learning! Keep forgiving yourself for being so hard on yourself, and remember: what we're accustomed to calling "mistakes" are really experiences to learn from.

In this book, I use the phrases "dying person," "sick person," and "patient" to avoid more convoluted wording. Inherent in these phrases are notions that hold us to old patterns. So remember: *We're all dying.* I don't believe there is such a thing as a "sick person"—only people with imbalances between their bodies, minds, feelings, and souls. "Patient" has an impersonal quality that denies our uniqueness and humanness, and promotes the illusion that a dying person's experience is separate from ours. Our experiences aren't separate. We aren't separate.

Come out of the circle of time and into
the circle of love.

—Rumi

1

THREE EXPERIENCES WITH DYING AT HOME

Friendship is a sheltering tree.

—Samuel Coleridge

I'd like to share with you my first experiences with dying at home. Although they take place in an earlier time in American cultural history, perhaps after reading them, dying at home won't seem like walking into the unknown. At least their stories will give you an idea of what it can be like. Their deaths, and each home death I have been privileged to share, were unique. And each was a story about love.

JOHN

John Muir was best known for the book he coauthored, *How to Keep Your Volkswagen Alive: A Manual of Step-by-Step Procedures for the Compleat Idiot.* What I remember most was his love, generosity, and the way he constantly heckled me to live in the present.

I met John and his wife, Eve, in the early 1970s in a colorful colonial town and artist colony in the high sierras of Guanajuato, Mexico. The big treat in San Miguel de Allende was Thursday afternoons at John and Eve's. There we soaked in the hot pool and talked and talked about our projects and dreams. John had a gift for sharing love and money to help his friends make their dreams come true without undermining their dignity or initiative.

Over the years, a loving family of friends grew. That family supported each of us in being and doing whatever we chose. Some wanted and needed a patriarch, so John allowed himself to be that patriarch. And he was a delightful one. He loved all the attention and had fun with the power, but at the same time, he encouraged us to take responsibility for ourselves and tried to teach us that "humans have evolved to where leaders are no longer necessary."

If a hero is someone who's true to his or her beliefs and inspires others, John was a hero. Physically, he looked the part. He was a huge, leonine, tawny-colored being with blue eyes that pierced outward appearances. John did and thought what he wanted, which ranged from the unique to the outrageous. Without regard for the traditional value of job security, he was at various times a musician, sailor, mechanic, welder, structural engineer, builder, and author. He was also a beatnik, hippie, philosopher, lover, husband, and father. He traveled the United States and Mexico in a converted thirty-three-passenger army bus and sailed a Chinese junk until it sank in a hurricane off Cape Hatteras.

When no publisher wanted the Volkswagen Idiot book, John and Eve had enough faith in it to sell a house and start their own publishing company. They made a reasonable fortune and shared it. Each January, John held a business meeting/party at a beach in Mexico and paid expenses for friends who otherwise couldn't have come to share their ideas and manuscripts.

John had an incessant curiosity about life. His second book, *The Velvet Monkey Wrench,* was a blueprint for a society based on an agreement among people to respect each other and the land. John and I became close amidst yelling, steaming, and reasoning as I helped edit it. Later, after we'd trekked through Nepal together, John continued to work on a book about the energy that gives life to matter, which he called "the life force."

John loved women, and there were generally lots around him. He felt we held a clue about this elusive life force. He knew it was connected to the balance of male and female energy in the universe. In his last couple of years, John was obsessed with his search to understand it. A number of friends asked him to take a break from the book because it seemed to be making him sick. But John wouldn't let go.

One hot June morning in Oregon in 1976, he stood up feeling dizzy after his usual three-minute headstand and fell. The dizziness continued and couldn't be diagnosed; a CAT scan showed nothing, and his ears and eyes were perfect. He asked Eve, seemingly out of the blue, "Is this just an inconvenience, or is this death?" By late August, the dizziness was worse, and his handwriting was shaky. A second CAT scan showed a growth on his brain. He decided on an operation, which verified a fast-growing malignant tumor, an offshoot of one in his lungs. The doctors gave him two months to two years. John was fifty-nine.

He recovered quickly from the operation and refused radiation therapy, joking, "If I'm wrong, will you dance on my grave?" Then he and Eve searched for alternative treatments and went camping in their favorite spots in the Southwest. Armed with laetrile, which some considered to be a hopeful alternative treatment at the time, they headed to Santa Fe, New Mexico. There, John tried acupuncture again, but he found it too painful. Except for occasional forays into ice cream, he stuck to a vegetable diet—a major change for a "meat and potatoes man." He denied having cancer and told us not to mention it. Every morning, he dictated his life force ideas into a tape recorder.

One day in mid-October, John woke up with a terrific headache. Pressure from the growing tumor was causing fluid to collect in his head. He agreed to have the fluid drained. This supposedly simple procedure impaired his speech. To a man who loved to talk, slurring his words was a kind of death. Blessedly, his thinking remained clear.

The doctors said if he stayed in the hospital, he'd be hooked up to life-support systems. After an exuberant session of playing guitars and singing "On the Bayou" and the old Leadbelly song "Pick a Bale of Cotton" around his hospital bed, it was obvious that his friends were too many and too noisy for a hospital. He wanted out. We wanted him out. Elizabeth, his friend and former wife, spoke for us all: "The quality of life is more important than the quantity," she said.

John and Eve didn't own a home in Santa Fe, so a friend lent them a large, empty adobe. In the four hours before the ambulance arrived with John, we made the house a home—rugs, pillows, wall hangings, rented TV and hospital bed, a complete kitchen, and a schedule for cooking and sitting with John in two-hour shifts. No one in particular directed. Each person sensed the needs and went about fulfilling them.

It was a glorious autumn afternoon in the Sangre de Cristo Mountains when the ambulance pulled up. John was carried on a stretcher through the open garden gate and down the stone path. The sun shone on him through golden aspen leaves. After we tucked him in bed next to a window partially opened to the fresh mountain air, he seemed relieved and content. Some of us fussed with food; others gathered around the fireplace and played guitars. Often, someone tiptoed in to see John sleeping, not because he needed checking on, just for the joy of seeing him at home.

That evening, we called John's friends from all over the country. "If you need to say good-bye to John in person," we said, "it's time to come." Already about twenty of us had gathered; eight lived in or camped around the house.

John orchestrated his dying as he did his living. Rusty, a nurse and masseur friend from Mexico, became coordinator for his needs. Some family members still had ideas about saving his body, and the first morning home, John said, "Let the kids test their theories." He believed actions are things to learn from. There are no mistakes, no being wrong. If we do nothing, we learn nothing. In fairness to the different treatments—vegetarian diet, laetrile, poultices, acupuncture, etc.—I believe that John tested them after he had already decided on some level to die.

One afternoon two friends put a clay poultice on John's neck and left him alone to play with a video camera in the living room. Everyone was making so much noise that no one heard John's bellow for help until after the poultice burned him. He was furious. "I want to see all of you with one of these on," he hollered.

My concern was preparing his soul for its voyage rather than attempting to save his body. I gave him Bach flower remedies—tinctures of flower essences that work on an energetic principle—which many believe help integrate the personality and the soul.

Day by day, I watched John and Eve as they decided what he did and did not want. Although he was very uncomfortable, he did not have severe pain. Perhaps the laetrile and Bach flower remedies had positive benefits in terms of pain control. It's hard to say, though, because according to the National Cancer Institute, 50–70 percent of cancer patients in treatment do not experience significant levels of pain. The percentage for those with advanced cancer is thirty, and 80–85 percent of the time the pain can be relieved.[1]

Within the family, loving factions developed over diet. Was it best to maintain an extreme cleansing diet, or was it too late for that? John wanted ice cream, not wheatgrass juice and raw vegetables. Seemed reasonable to me. Ice cream and cigarettes were sneaked to him to protect the feelings of friends not yet ready for him to die.

In some ways, I was one of those not-yet-ready people. One night, a friend of John and Eve's brought her drunk and suicidal brother to the house and left him there while she went dancing. I was outraged. "How can anyone be so thoughtless?" I asked. "John is dying in the next room!" But Eve didn't seem bothered. Without words, she helped me understand that there was enough love for everyone. It was an important lesson for me about operating from a belief in plenty instead of scarcity. Even still, it took me a while to let go of my anger.

Time seemed to stand still as we shared those last few weeks together. When we weren't massaging, bathing, feeding, or just being with John, we sat around the fire, reminisced and shared experiences, and caught up on current news. In the evening, some made a circle of power for healing around him, and some chanted. A Native American medicine man was called, and he made a "helping the spirit to leave" ceremony. A minister from the Native American Church, who'd married John and Eve ten years earlier, came to give his blessing. An oncologist, two unconventional MDs, and a homeopath came in and out. Two couples who weren't speaking to each other gracefully and with difficulty laid aside their grievances. Several of us had opportunities to examine jealousy or irritation as we imagined that so-and-so was "more important" or "taking over."

There was, however, one thought we all shared. What would the family be like without John? We wondered why he was dying when he seemed to live with such joy and enthusiasm. Our theories about his death likely revealed more about our relationship with him and about our own beliefs than about the actual reasons for his death. I believe John and I had the same "dis-ease": an attachment to being in control and a resistance to surrendering. We were both stubborn, and we were both looking for answers outside of ourselves.

Later, I came to understand John's dying as his ultimate lesson in surrender. Without surrender, the feminine principle, he couldn't complete his ideas on the life force. If we haven't learned it earlier, dying can teach us to surrender. When we surrender, we open to the life force that is always within us. Perhaps John wanted the answer to his question so much that he created his dying to get the answer.

After it seemed obvious to us that saving his body was impossible, John seemed to be deciding whether to fight or let go, surrender to death. Some of us were reading Elisabeth Kübler-Ross's description of the stages of dying: denial, isolation, anger, bargaining, depression, and acceptance. John moved back and forth between all of them. Most of the time, he denied he was dying; this left him in control but unable to find ways to heal himself. "Let me just finish the book," he bargained, or, "Oh, okay, if Eve and I can just take a trip to Hawaii first." Off and on, he was depressed. "I was always afraid of being hurt," he said, "and now I hurt."

It was difficult to talk with John about dying because he hadn't accepted that it was happening to him. He'd often said, "Death is the greatest adventure of them all. I'll see what it's like when I get there." But now, he was angry at dying. Yet being angry and fighting seemed to clear the air so he could finally accept his dying. Once he did, it took him only a day and a half to die.

Occasionally, images of that time still come to me: Eve's graceful calm and humor; the oncologist in suit and tie crossing paths in John's room with a medicine man in a black-feathered hat; Eve lifting cupped hands of new-fallen snow to John so he could enjoy the first snowfall; the two of them cuddling in the narrow hospital bed; Eve and Elizabeth working side by side to bathe him; John watching Walter Cronkite report the news with me while Eve was off dancing; John telling everyone who brought up business, "Look, my will's in order and if you don't leave me alone, I'll put Star and Craig in charge of everything." Both sons were eighteen. Earlier he'd said he wanted the "sixty-peso funeral," the cheapest in Mexico!

The last weekend, there were fewer people, and we all stayed overnight in the house on Victoria Street that had become our home. The whisperings in the kitchen subsided. It was quiet and peaceful. John was tending to dying, and each of us to finishing our "business" with him.

The day before he died, John asked Dr. Greg if there was any way for him to live. "No," said Greg, "we can only make you as comfortable as possible without making you unconscious."

"I'm too uncomfortable to go on living anyway," John said.

Then, as soon as Greg left the room, John said to me, "Deborah, you've got to stop your compulsive lying."

That stopped me in my tracks. John still had a knack for getting someone's attention by using something they were attached to—like my image of myself as an honest person. At first, I thought he was referring to my saying "nobody dies," because the doctor had just told him he was going to die. But I realized that wasn't it. I felt stunned, kicked in the gut. I asked him to repeat what he said, and he did. "Don't you dare die without explaining to me what you mean," I said, choked and teary. "It's not fair to leave a ghost like that."

"Stop saying you're *going to* quit smoking or *going to* do anything in the future," he said. What I understood from his slurred words was that he was trying to help me stop setting booby traps for myself. Often enough, he'd witnessed me project something I *might* do *in the future,* then feel like I was a failure when I didn't do it. One of his last gifts to me was trying again to help me live in the *present.*

That night none of us expected John to live until the morning. We held our last healing circle. This time the healing was for John, not for his body. He seemed to finally accept that we loved *him,* not just the part of him that helped us out or made our lives happier. We loved him whether or not he finished his book.

After the healing circle he said, "Eve, I love you...such good friends." And someone said, "You've been a wonderful friend to us." John did not speak again.

We scheduled ourselves by twos every two hours to help him sit up and cough. Now his breathing had an unnerving rattling sound. He couldn't swallow and we kept moistening his parched lips. It was terrible to watch helplessly as he suffered. Only later did I understand that his soul, or consciousness, was already out of the body. The body was suffering, but John was not suffering.

The shifts shortened to one hour, then to half an hour. When not on shift, we cuddled together like children and slept on mattresses covering the living room floor. I remember looking down on my sleeping partners and feeling how much I loved them.

John's body labored all night, coughing and struggling for air. The body seemed to have a life of its own, and it hung on.

In the morning I went to my construction job plastering adobe houses. Dealing with my feelings was not as easy as smoothing bumps on walls. My heart and mind were with John and the family. Each time I called home, John was still alive. After work I stopped by the most expensive grocery store in Santa Fe and brought two baskets of fresh raspberries and a Toblerone chocolate bar. Perhaps outer nourishment might ease the inner loss. I ate one whole basket on the way home and saved the other for Eve.

When I got home, John was weaker and Eve was away. She'd gone out in her car to yell and cry. This, along with dancing, usually helped her remain calm. This time she came back mad. "John has pulled us into a terrible sadness trip. He said death is the greatest adventure—he might as well relax and enjoy it!" Gently she repeated this to John. He relaxed and breathed easier. Maybe he'd been waiting to hear from her that it was okay to let go.

She left the room and we sat there and ate the Toblerone. A few minutes later, Rusty motioned me to bring her back. Eve came and held John's hand. At three o'clock in the afternoon, John stopped breathing. The six of us there chanted "om" as he left his body. Om, or *Aum,* is understood by many as the Primal Sound that connects us to everything. It's used particularly by Hindus and Buddhists.

Tears of sadness, relief, and joy rolled down our waiting faces. We held each other and prayed, each in his or her own way, for his soul to move on quickly. We lit candles and incense. Then we dressed John's body in his favorite blue flannel shirt and a pair of Eve's drawstring pants. His own were now too big. Eve put an *Ojo de Dios* (God's Eye) at his head and a child's pinwheel in his hand. Rusty shaved him. John's face seemed to fill out; all signs of pain and struggle were gone. His real nobility of heart was again visible in the old familiar face.

That night we cried and laughed and told stories. I'd be talking with someone with tears running down my face and the next minute we'd both be laughing as we greeted others. Someone on her way to the house when John died said she saw him whooping up and down the foothills on a roller coaster laughing his head off. Friends phoned and were phoned. Eve called Wavy Gravy, an old activist friend who founded Camp Winarainbow, a summer camp that uses circus skills to teach kids about themselves and life. When she told him about John's death, his reply was, "Well...it was Patrick Henry's second choice!"

Two friends went off with a bottle of Scotch to build a coffin and hammer a thumb. The burial laws in New Mexico are very humane. You may bury someone on private property within twenty-four hours of death if the site is at least fifty feet from water. You file a burial certificate and get a body transfer permit—a one-stop operation. Later you note the burial site on the land deed so a highway or something isn't built over the grave. Friends offered a weedy little field by their house as a burial site. We decided to plant an orchard there.

The next morning, waiting for the coffin to arrive, many of us felt a little unfocused, like the day after Christmas. We wanted to bury him quickly. We'd had plenty of time to "clear" with John, and it was time to move on. I went to buy a cherry tree and a Jonathan apple for the new orchard and flowers for the grave. We arranged for a truck; a hearse didn't feel right. When it finally arrived, we realized our impression that John was a giant of a man had manifested in a ridiculously large, nine-foot by four-foot coffin. We placed John's body on a faded red *serape.* It was a relief to be outside. The body had begun to smell, which wasn't as noticeable outside. (I learned later that the smell was probably from body fluids released after death.)

We followed the truck with the coffin over to Ken and Barb's field. Sawhorses to support the coffin were set up under a clear early winter sky. People came and looked and cried. Some put treasures in the box they wanted to send with John's body: copies of his two books, a piece of jade, a bit of lapis lazuli, a Tibetan *mandala,* dancing shoes. Another writer put his pen in John's shirt pocket. "You can't put an author away without a pen," he said.

We dug a great hole in the earth, much deeper than needed. Nearly everyone wanted a turn digging. I watched a friend with tears running down his face work with a pick and shovel until he was exhausted. "This is the last thing I can do for him," he said. It was great therapy to be out in the fresh air using our bodies. I wondered later why people let professionals take this therapy away from them.

We made a large circle, some sixty people, and joined hands around the coffin. Whoever wanted to could speak. Eve had asked a friend to read a passage from *The Velvet Monkey Wrench.*

> *Imitating someone else's style just because they are stronger, richer, fatter, or hipper is a stone drag. Picking our very own lifestyle is not a process of copying.*

Not many of us trusted that if we opened our mouths words would come. Instead we sang "When the Saints Go Marching In," and two women sat on a knoll playing a French horn and a fiddle. Eve tossed a yellow rose on top of the box for an absent friend as it was lowered into the earth. We shoveled in the earth and planted and watered a Jonathan apple tree.

A friend was freed, and a new orchard begun. It was a great day to celebrate, with feasting, talking, dancing, crying, holding, and being held. Someone asked, "Why aren't we this close all the time?"

John's last gift was to bring us together and give us an opportunity to learn that "Dying is okay."

MARY

My next experience with dying came not quite a year later in Santa Fe, while we were still discussing writing a book about the last one. What we'd learned with John seemed useful to share.

Mary Conley's dying was very different from John's. Cancer was about the only thing they had in common. Mary had few close friends and almost no money. Her wealth was her faith that death is a doorway to more life. The richness of our shared faith, my experience with John, and fewer people to orchestrate made her dying much easier for me.

There were four of us: Mary, her twenty-one-year-old son Craig, myself, and later Craig's friend Jean. At first we felt alone, a tiny island tending to dying in a world going about business as usual.

Our combined resources at the time were two hundred dollars and a house with one month's rent paid. Neither Craig nor Jean had been in close contact with someone dying, although Mary's husband (Craig's father) had died ten years earlier of cancer. Mary's daughter in Mexico had already coped with what she could and wasn't with us. That seemed okay. Each person has to decide what's right for them when someone's dying; not everyone has to be or can be present.

Mary and I met in San Miguel about the same time I met John and Eve, and we became close spiritual sisters. After her husband died, she traveled with her children and continued to study astrology and metaphysics. When we met, she was a doting young grandmother often caring for her baby granddaughter by herself while writing a book on Tarot. The Tarot is an ancient divination system that uses universal archetypal symbols on cards to bring the unconscious mind to our awareness.

When I was especially happy or depressed, I'd head down the cobblestone alleys to Mary's tiny adobe house at the bottom of the hill. Regardless of my emotional state when I arrived, I always left feeling better and seeing my life more clearly. Many others can say the same. Mary shared herself and her wisdom with whomever arrived on her doorstep and wanted to receive it.

For two years, almost no one knew Mary had cancer. During the second year, she was housemother in a home for pregnant teenagers in Albuquerque, New Mexico. Mary was the one to hold a rejected girl's hand as she went through labor. Her love and guidance helped at least thirty young girls live through and learn from a potentially fearful experience. And at the same time she worked on healing her own dis-ease.

To Mary, cancer was a teacher, and she looked for the lessons it offered. She understood life as a spiral of births into flesh and deaths into spirit, moving closer each time to one's God self. Cancer was helping her learn something she needed to understand for this journey home. Mary believed it was about the fear and unworthiness she'd felt growing up without parents.

Since childhood, she'd struggled between the two parts of her personality that she called Pitiful Pearl and Mary C. Pitiful Pearl was always afraid and felt she didn't deserve anything good from life. Mary C., on the other hand, was wise and courageous, and manifested herself strongly when Mary worked as a housemother. Mary thought that as Mary C. got stronger, Pitiful Pearl felt threatened and expressed herself by creating illness. It seemed to me that not expressing her sadness nor loving herself as generously as she loved others were important factors in her illness. Until the last five months, she seemed to have eliminated the cancer.

For me, Mary's dying began with a phone call I received while visiting my parents in Texas. Craig said he and Mary were alone in her tiny second-story apartment in Albuquerque and were both feeling crazy with the confinement and summer heat. They'd just returned from trips to a clinic in Mexico and to a psychic healer in Costa Rica, and Mary was in terrible shape.

"Okay," I told Craig, "I'm coming. We'll go to my house in Santa Fe." After I said it, I was assailed by doubts. "How can I care for her and work on my master's thesis and make enough money to survive? What if she's in terrible pain and I can't help? Where will I move if I have to leave my house because the echoes of her pain haunt me?"

In Albuquerque, I found a tiny, shriveled being who couldn't move or eat alone. When I'd last seen Mary five months earlier, she was a very attractive, peppery-red-haired woman of fifty who looked forty. Now she appeared a gray, skeletal eighty. My initial joy at seeing her changed to shock and pain. My chest felt like it was pushed against my spine. Knowing I needed time and space to grieve, I suggested I go to Santa Fe, clean house, and then return for her.

During the hour-long drive home, I yelled from as deep in my gut as I could. Yelling relived the pressure, and I was free to race around preparing the four small rooms. I chose the living room for Mary, because afternoon sunlight illuminated it and the mountains, and because I needed the nourishing morning light of my bedroom. I moved furniture, hung a wind chime and birdfeeder outside the living room windows, bought a bedpan and straws that bent, washed and ironed peach silk nightgowns, rented a wheelchair and potty chair, and chose music she might like.

We couldn't afford an ambulance, so we decided to bring Mary to Santa Fe in my pickup truck. Craig called the Fire Department Rescue Squad to carry her down the steep stairs of her apartment. They helped Mary onto the foam mattress in the pickup, and we wedged her in with quilts and pillows. Because Craig's truck was threatening to break down, I followed him slowly up the valley between the Jemez and Sangre de Christo (Blood of Christ) mountains. The trip was horrendous, but Mary, with her usual grace, said, "Oh, it was just fine. Thank God to be home in the mountains."

Somehow we got her from the pickup to the house to the bed. As we got her settled in, I felt again the blessed relief I'd felt when John came home. Now Mary was home and comfortable and had two people who loved her to do whatever was needed. The house was peaceful, filled with loving new energy and enormous bouquets of wild gold sunflowers.

Craig was exhausted. He'd dropped out the first quarter of his senior year of college to be with his mother. For six weeks he had single-handedly fed, bathed, and moved her everywhere (even between countries), and had helped her with whatever she'd needed, including enemas. Knowing he could sleep soundly for the first time in months was deeply satisfying to me. He had to sleep on a sheepskin rug in the prayer room, but at least there was someone else to take a turn.

There was no hospice in Santa Fe in those days. Because we had almost no money, we set about phoning everyone in town we could think of for help. If an agency or office couldn't help, we asked if they knew who could. We followed every lead. In a few days we had laetrile and two offers of wheelchairs to replace the rented one. We found a visiting nurse service that had a government grant to help the terminally ill. They supported our decision to be at home, sent gentle, competent nurses to visit twice a week, and said we could call them at any time.

I knew of another group, Open Hands, who visited with the elderly, disabled, and terminally ill and provided counseling and other services like running errands, bathing, cooking, or just companionship. They'd take over for us if we needed it. We found that Mary was eligible for Social Security and applied on her behalf, although the money did not arrive until after she died. We found a county emergency medical fund that would pay any hospital expenses. Shanti, a volunteer counseling group, was willing to send a counselor. The nurse friend who helped us when John was dying gave Mary shots and didn't charge us.

Dr. Greg visited Mary, took care of her the night she went to the hospital, and never sent a bill. He even took me to dinner one night when I had to get away. Another friend co-signed a bank loan so I could splurge on a color TV. With a TV, Mary could have some variety and diversion when she wanted, and I felt freer to do what I wanted. I went to a flower shop and told the florist that my friend was dying, that

I wanted to surround her with beauty, and that I didn't have much money. He would let me rifle through the trash cans where the imperfect flowers are tossed, and I'd go home happily with bouquets of yellow roses and delicate white baby's breath.

Our day-to-day supporters were each other, God, and Gathanna. The Quimby Center in Alamogordo, New Mexico, and the White Lodge in England sent spiritual healing and support. One friend came with food, massages, love, and recipes. One of my biggest fears had been what to cook. Another friend gave me energy by calling to check on how I was doing. Craig's relatives sent love and money, and I sold antique clothing off the back porch.

I was surprised by how much joy I could find in that little house with my friend dying in the living room. For a few minutes each morning before getting out of bed, I meditated on joy and imagined myself as the "joyful servant." I put signs that read "JOY" on the refrigerator door and over my bed to remind me of it throughout the day. As I nurtured my joyful servant, I experienced more and more of what a privilege it was to share this opportunity to learn with Mary.

I found joy in our talks, watching the birds, dabbing on Tea Rose perfume, hearing the wind chime, and massaging her. There was joy in our jokes about our spiritual interests or about my using her as an excuse to get out of meetings I didn't want to attend. There was joy in waltzing—when Mary couldn't walk alone anymore, and I had to hold her up under her arms, I'd ask, "Madame, may I have this waltz?" Our silliness let her know she wasn't a burden and, I imagine, helped her release some of the frustration of no longer being able to walk alone.

I took time for myself—for Tai Chi, jogging, paperwork, and gardening—and encouraged Craig to do the same. He and Jean went camping for two days and visited with old friends. At twenty-one, Craig and Jean seemed young to be going through this. I would have felt motherly, except they were so sensitive and capable.

Even though we were receiving all this amazing support, and Mary was taking her increasing limitations mostly in stride, she was still in denial about her impending death. The denial continued for about three weeks: Maybe if she took more enzymes, she would throw off the cancer. Maybe a piece of stool, and not a tumor, was blocking her intestines. Maybe we should put poultices on the huge lump on her leg and open and drain it so it wouldn't poison her body. She needed hope, but she was looking for it in the wrong place; she was still too focused on saving her body.

One day Mary decided she wanted a coffee enema to detoxify her liver, which would hopefully eliminate the cancer. (Coffee enemas are sometimes used in alternative cancer treatments to help detoxify the liver, but must be part of a larger healing program.) The plan was to build a bench in my white prayer room and give her the enemas there, close to the bathroom. I hit the wall! I couldn't stand the idea of my sanctuary being messed up, and I felt guilty for it. "Deborah, how can you be so persnickety!" I railed at myself. "Those enemas might help Mary live. At least they'd support her trying to help herself!" I wasn't compassionate enough with myself to think, "There's something important to me about this prayer room, something that gives me the strength to support Mary through this experience."

To assuage my guilt about my "selfishness," I suggested an alternative plan: a liver flush commonly used in holistic healing. It's a cocktail of cayenne, garlic, ginger, olive oil, and lemon juice mixed in orange juice to help it down. I mixed one up, a little heavy on the cayenne, and gave it to Mary. She took two sips, gagged, and said, "It's awful!" And in five minutes she was shaking, sweating, and delirious. I jumped into the bed and held her, thinking, "Deborah, she's going to die. You've killed her." Fortunately for me she didn't die, but I felt guilty anyway. I hadn't yet graduated from the school of guilt.

About a week before Mary died, lumps sprouted all over her body. It was obvious she was dying, yet she was still denying it. Craig often felt disgusted and angry with his mother's lack of acceptance. "She's denying everything she ever taught me," he'd say. He wished it was already over and felt guilty for wishing it. He didn't know that many people living with someone they love who is dying slowly have similar feelings. I suggested it was perfectly natural, that his guilt was unnecessary. It's possible to feel "I wish it were over" and have compassion at the same time. For my part, sometimes I was fed up and wanted Mary to be somewhere, mentally, that she wasn't: accepting of her death. But my non-acceptance was my problem, not hers.

Dealing with our frustrations was more difficult than physically caring for Mary. We'd sit on the back porch, watching the chipmunks play, and talk out the things that bothered us. Sharing our fear, sadness, and frustration helped release those emotions.

After one back porch discussion, Craig and I decided to tell Mary what we thought about her condition. We were frustrated with the increasingly desperate attempts to save her. Dr. Greg wasn't around to do the talking for us, so I told Mary, "We feel it would take a miracle to save your body. We believe in miracles, and it would have to be a big one...soon." This left *some* room for hope and gave her a clear picture of what *we* thought was happening.

Still, she decided on a trip to the hospital to find out if some physical or mechanical obstruction other than a cancerous tumor was what was preventing her from eating and eliminating. Although we didn't think much of the idea, it wasn't *our* life, so we arranged it. This time we had to use an ambulance. The four of us spent one night in the hospital.

When we came home, Mary had to decide whether or not to continue the intravenous feedings that kept her body from dehydrating. Dr. Greg told her what he knew about dehydration. She decided not to continue the IVs, a decision that took great courage. In saying "no," she was also saying "I know I'm going to die." She chose, in effect, to die of dehydration instead of cancer. It's not a bad way to go. You slip slowly into unconsciousness and the main discomfort is dryness in the mouth.

Once Mary accepted that she was dying, her depression ended. We could talk about death and what her work might be on the other side. She told us that, if possible, she would report to us. We decided her sign for communicating with us after death would be sunflowers. If we were meditating and saw a sunflower, whatever we heard would be from Mary. After her death, I received a couple of sunflower messages.

Three days before she died, Mary said, "Get ready for Sunday. I'll be leaving." One part of me was irritated. For months I'd planned a retreat in the mountains that weekend with Patricia Sun, a spiritual teacher and healer. It took a while for me to realize that a much more important spiritual learning opportunity was going on in my own home. We started to get ready.

I suggested that Craig talk with his mother about anything unclear in their relationship so he wouldn't be left with the "I wish I hads." Mary's daughter called from Mexico, and I held the phone. It was a privilege to share that conversation: a mother saying good-bye to a daughter with whom she had not had an easy relationship, expressing her love and her understanding of her daughter's absence.

Craig had Mary's land transferred to his name to avoid lawyers later. Mary had a few other material possessions and told Craig what to do with them. She gave me the perfect reminder of our common commitment: a little gold Florentine box with the Prayer of Saint Francis, the same prayer Mother Teresa later sent me.

I've often wondered how Craig felt as he went to the lumber yard to buy pine boards and quietly set about building a box for his mother on the back porch. He put his heart and hands into making the best box he could, using screws instead of nails so Mary wouldn't hear the hammering. I became the "interior decorator" and for our sake made the inside of the box beautiful with old hand-sewn quilts.

Saturday and Sunday we let out the stops—no more pacing ourselves. At night we slept lightly in my room, with the door open so we could hear her calls or changes in breathing. During the day we were with her constantly. Seven or eight times daily we massaged her back, hands, and feet. Touching was among the few things she still enjoyed. It was important for her to know that we weren't too repulsed to touch her lump-covered body. We continued to wash her teeth, bathe her, and comb her hair. To alleviate the dryness in her mouth, we used ice chips or held a wet washcloth for her to suck on.

Sunday, while we were practicing sliding a suction tube down the throat of the visiting nurse in case we'd need this procedure, Mary's breathing became very heavy and labored. I thought she was leaving and suggested she move toward the Light and practice letting go. After hardly speaking for two days, she managed to get out, "You're rushing me."

We broke up laughing and joked about the rebellion on our hands. Who is to know God's timetable or what unfinished work she had to do on a level beyond our understanding? From that point on, she was in and out of consciousness.

She mumbled or mimed to us to turn her in bed about every twenty minutes, which was tiring because she couldn't help at all. Because she couldn't move, eat, or drink, and her skin was raw, she was in extreme discomfort. We asked if she wanted a shot of Demerol that had been prescribed, and she nodded. Earlier we'd practiced in the kitchen giving shots to a helpless orange. Jean was elected to give Mary the first one because of her greater experience—giving shots to mice in a biology lab. Because Jean and Craig were willing, I didn't have to face my fear of shots...this time.

In the beginning, we'd been afraid that we might not know what to do for Mary, but as each situation arose, we found we could handle it, which increased our confidence for the next. Taking care of things ourselves seemed preferable to waiting for a nurse.

Demerol was the first pain medication Mary took since way back when she could swallow an occasional Tylenol. In the hospital, doctors and nurses were amazed she wasn't in pain. She had tumors throughout her body, and her vital organs were barely functioning.

Monday evening Dr. Greg stopped by and said, "You know she could go on breathing like this for a couple of days." I crumbled. A few nights earlier he had gently and sensitively repeated the now familiar words, "We can't save your body, but we'll make you as comfortable as possible." Because we'd stopped pacing ourselves, I was exhausted and didn't know if I could keep going as long as she could. We decided I'd go to dinner with Greg, and the next morning Craig and Jean would go for a walk in the hills.

As much as I needed to get away, I didn't enjoy it. I felt divided; half of me wanted to be with Mary. When I got home after midnight, Craig and Jean were just lying down on the floor to rest. "How's it going?" I asked. "We just sat quietly with Mom all evening," Craig said. "She's the same." I went in to see her. She was still breathing but looked dead already. I said offhandedly, "She looks macabre," and went into the bathroom. Craig called, and she was gone before I got back to her room. Perhaps she'd been waiting for me to get home so Craig and Jean wouldn't be alone.

We stood shocked for a bit by death, the event we'd been anticipating. While it was sinking in, I distracted myself by phoning Greg to tell him Mary was dead and to remember the death certificate. Calmed, I went back to her room. We lit candles, said prayers for her to be on her way, and held each other. Then we dressed her in a favorite peach silk and lace nightgown. I tied a scarf under her chin to the top of her head (as if she had a toothache) so her mouth would set closed.

With the focus of our energy suddenly gone, we felt shaky, uncertain. Holding each other and praying helped steady us. We all thought of food at the same time and left the body to go rummage through the refrigerator. How surprising it was to be hungry! We talked awhile, and then fell into our sleeping places, feeling we could sleep forever.

Greg woke us at 6:00 a.m. to certify her dead. I could easily have waited till 9:00 to have the obvious made official. We lifted Mary's body into the coffin, which, after all my warnings about John's absurdly big one, seemed to me a little snug. Craig maintained it was "just right." After putting in her Tarot deck, Craig hammered down the top of the box, and he and a childhood friend, Joey, loaded the heavy coffin into my pickup. We were to meet Greg at the Office of Vital Statistics to fill out the death certificate and body transport form. Mary wanted to be buried on her land in the mountains three hours north of Santa Fe.

Greg thought our digging crew was understaffed and volunteered to help, but not without breakfast. So while Craig, Joey, and Jean set off with borrowed picks and shovels, I had breakfast with Greg. The young doctor said, "I hope if I help enough folks, there'll be people around to give me a good burial some day."

On the way, I stopped at my usual gas station. The owner asked, "What ya up to today?" I answered, "I'm off to the mountains to bury my friend," and motioned toward the back of the truck. The look on his face when he saw the coffin delighted me. Our relationship was different after that day; he took a special interest in what I carried in the back of my truck.

It was an exquisite late summer day. The high desert country was covered with purple asters, golden chamisa, and silver Indian sage. We chose a spot called The Meadow that overlooks valleys and more mountains. "Meadow" in the Southwest generally means "open," not green and grassy. This one was covered with gray, weathered wood, sculpted like driftwood. As we dug, Greg took the role of "the one who knows." I let go and was silly—and how I needed to be silly.

I shoveled a little, but mostly walked in the wind and felt the joy of being free in the mountains after so many days indoors. The others joked and told stories; they dug and rested, ate food and drank beer. The hole seemed to get shallower instead of deeper. I kept singing, "Bury me four feet deep in the lone prairie!" Meanwhile, Craig wanted the hole to be the standard "six feet deep." He insisted, "The hole has to be deep enough so animals can't dig her up." Even though this was unlikely, his need needed to be respected.

When the sun began to set and we were still digging, I became worried. I was due back in town for a lecture I was co-sponsoring. Cell phones had not yet been invented, and there was nothing to do but let go and trust that someone would handle it. We finished digging in the headlight beams of the pickups with the moon already up.

I lashed together a cross of four equal arms and placed it in a circle of stones. As a handful of earth ran through my fingers, the sense of loss of a sister caught up with me. I cried. Greg squatted beside me and repeated a Navajo prayer:

May it be beautiful before me.
May it be beautiful behind me.
May it be beautiful below me.
May it be beautiful above me.
May it be beautiful all around me.
In beauty it is finished.

DAD

While I was writing the first edition of this book, I knew my father was dying. My friends' deaths and writing this book were part of my preparation to accept his death.

Other than having to move a lot because Dad had been a military officer, my family was quite ordinary. We loved each other, and we were fiercely loyal. When we found out we had cancer, we did not see it as Dad's alone, but as the concern of us all.

It was Easter time, and the bluebonnets were blooming when we gathered in San Antonio, Texas, to be with him for his first surgery. We were frightened. When hours and more hours passed and we were still sitting in a waiting room at the VA hospital, we knew the cancer must be more extensive than the surgeons had thought.

Dad came out of surgery into a ward with exceptionally overworked nurses, which made them appear incompetent and unloving. The ward he shared with three other men was like a TV M.A.S.H. unit. The humor in the situation saved us. We were all in the same leaky lifeboat together!

The chief instigator, a man named Dolph, wore a panama hat with his pajamas, sneaked cigarettes, and drank hot coffee right before his temperature was taken. Anything except pain medications that the men needed, we had to do or find. We'd go off "midnight requisitioning," looking through closets for pajamas, sheets, towels, ice. Stolen lemon swabs were the pièce de résistance!

The camaraderie of the four men—a Navy admiral's steward, an army master sergeant, a warrant officer, and my father, a colonel—helped us adjust to his situation. At times we laughed so hard that Dad literally had to hold his stitches to keep them from bursting. And the laughter opened our hearts and dissolved some of the pain and fear.

After surgery, Dad's way to treat colon cancer was chemotherapy. That was not my way. I'd studied and worked with natural healing and had seen friends heal themselves of cancer without drugs and surgery. Choosing chemotherapy seemed to me, at that time, like signing a death warrant, because it severely damages the body's immune system. I knew Dad had to do it his own way, but I didn't want him to die! I gave him all the information I had on alternative healing and his response was, "I don't want to be the world's greatest cancer expert." He had faith in the medical system he grew up with and in a young Dr. Page at the VA hospital. The VA hospital was connected to the University of Texas Medical School and the MD Anderson Cancer Center. One week each month he stayed in the hospital for chemotherapy.

I returned to Santa Fe furious with the medical establishment, which admitted it didn't have the answer but insinuated that its way was the only way. I was furious with the army for sending human beings, including my father, to be guinea pigs at the nuclear bomb tests in Nevada in the 1950s. I was angry with everything and I hurt. There were lots of summer mornings when I sat on my back porch eating breakfast with tears rolling into my cereal. Slowly, very slowly, what I knew in my head entered my heart: each of us has to live and die in our own way. I began to take interest in my work again.

I thought of Dad often that summer as I worked on this book. I remembered him as a father. I remembered he and Mom tucking the twins, Judy and Suzy, and me into bed every night; his singing a song to wake us up for school; his taking me alone to Holland, braiding my pigtails, and letting me pick as many tulips as I wanted; teaching us to shoot and hunt; taking us exploring on the weekends, even when we didn't want to go. I remembered his face at the airport as I looked up at him from a wheelchair when he met me and my sheepdog in Mexico after I came home sick from the diplomatic service in Chile. I remembered his voice when, some years later, I phoned from Mexico to say I'd broken my back, and later he and Mom took turns visiting me twice a day in the hospital in San Antonio. I remembered the way he helped me up and down the halls as I learned to walk again. I remembered his wanting to go to New England with Mom to help Suzy when her first child, Joshua, was born, and instead staying home to take care of my sheepdog. He loved us, trusted us, and was proud of us. The only real gripe I remember was when he used to say, "Do it right or don't do it at all," and "right" meant "his way."

Who was this man I loved so much? He was my mother's husband for forty-three years. But that's her story. What I know is the light from their marriage gave other people strength.

Col. Edward Duda was an army officer for thirty years. (My friends would say, "But how can an army officer be so mellow?") What was it like for him after he retired as chief of staff of an army base, accustomed to telling twenty thousand men when to jump, when Mom would tell him, "Put your dishes on the left side of the sink"? Who was this quiet, charming man who reminded some of Jimmy Stewart (which secretly delighted me)? I'd watch him and wonder. He once even said, "I wish you wouldn't watch me so much."

Dad was born a few years after his parents arrived steerage class on a boat from Poland. My grandfather worked hard as a house painter to make it in a new country. However, when my dad was a child, being part of an ethnic group wasn't fashionable, which meant he grew up wanting to be an American, not a Polack kid. I think he was embarrassed that his parents didn't speak better English, and he never learned to speak Polish. He constantly sought to prove a Duda was as good as a Johnson, Jones, or Smith. Because American culture values doing and achieving, he set out to achieve: editor of the yearbook, captain of the track team, the fastest runner ("The Irvington Flash"), senior class president, the Zippity Duda who worked his way through college and graduated with honors.

First the Depression, then World War II, made Dad and nearly everyone else think about security. He was called into the army the day after I was born, liked it, and stayed. He expected to be a general, and his buddies, who became Chiefs of Staff of the Australian, British, and Israeli armies, expected he would become Chief of Staff of the U.S. Army. But the army, like every company, has its politics, and he didn't make it. We were proud of him anyway, but I know it hurt.

Especially in the beginning, I was plagued by the questions "Why cancer? Why him?" He was such a quiet, peaceful man. What in his emotional nature contributed to his dis-ease?

One evening we recorded Dad's life story up to his high school years. One of the first things he remembered was an accident when he was seven. He was relaxed and having fun when a kid hit him in the eye with a baseball bat. "From then on"' he said, "my vision was distorted." Later he related, "When I was a boy, I believed the most important thing was being in control; if I wasn't, I got hurt. My family got upset when I was hurt. I grew up believing that my being hurt made others suffer...so when I hurt, I kept it to myself. I kept swallowing the hurt. When I was older, I didn't hurt anymore...I wouldn't let myself. But still, things happened that hurt and it just sat inside. I picked up the radiation in Nevada but without all the hurt, it wouldn't have affected me. The hurt was a weakness the radiation could attach itself to...the hurt became the cancer."

As a little girl I saw the hurt and decided I had to be Dad's protectress, and now he had cancer and I couldn't protect him. Part of me still wanted to, and part of me realized this was his opportunity to learn.

That summer and fall, everything went along fairly smoothly. Mom sent out Christmas cards that said, "We have cancer and we're doing fine." We all wondered if this was the last year Dad would put the somewhat scruffy white angel we'd had for thirty-five years on top of the tree.

One morning four months later, when I was visiting Mexico, I woke up knowing something was wrong at home and telephoned. Mom was crying. Dad was in the hospital again. They'd found a huge tumor in his liver and spots on his lungs and were planning to operate. On top of the shock of being told Dad's cancer was spreading, she'd been sitting up all the previous night alone in the house with my dying sheepdog, Benjy, in her lap. When I called, she'd just returned from taking him to the vet to be euthanized.

After a series of painful tests, the doctors decided Dad's tumor was inoperable. They decided to insert a tube into his liver so chemotherapy drugs could be fed directly into it, which they said was "a minor operation." Mom was holding together pretty well. She'd always said, "I can do anything I have to."

I arrived home in time for the surgery. In the waiting room, Mom played cards, I meditated and sent love to Dad, and we picnicked on fried chicken. The ward room held a strange fascination for me. I watched deserted old and young soldiers sitting in wheelchairs, connected to tubes, many with mechanical voice boxes, watching TV quiz shows, while life slowly drained out of them. I remembered Mother Teresa calling loneliness the worst human disease, and I imagined each man filled with love. When I focused on love, I worried less about Dad.

When I saw orderlies wheeling him, writhing in pain, toward his room on a stretcher, I ran into the hall. That old instinct to protect him welled up, and I could do nothing.

After Dad came home, we buried Benjy's ashes in the backyard. Dad cried and cried—for himself, for Benjy, for us all. It was the first time I'd seen him cry since he'd found out he had cancer, although Mom said they'd had some good cries together.

Each day we had to flush a solution through the tube in the artery to Dad's liver. If we didn't clamp the tube properly, blood would spurt out all over. After working in the hospital, this didn't frighten me. For Mom and Dad it was very unnerving at first. Taking responsibility for irrigating that tube was an important step in increasing their confidence that they could take care of Dad's needs at home.

The talk at home changed from "Can he be cured?" to "How long might he live?" Dad hoped to make it to hunting season and Christmas. Together he and I were learning what Mom seemed born knowing: surrender. Instead of learning it from my friends with their seemingly free lifestyles, I was learning it from this modest middle-class couple who lived in the suburbs. Dad accepted he was dying nearly a year before he died, so he was able to live fully in his remaining time. But even after he accepted what was happening, it took him a while to get used to not being in control.

I returned to New Mexico to continue writing. Suzy and her boys moved to Texas to live with Mom and Dad. Because Dad had chosen chemotherapy, I prepared myself to hear that he'd chosen to die in a hospital. Also, Mom, Suzy, and Judy had all said they didn't think they could handle his dying at home. Finally, even I could accept that dying in a hospital was okay.

In October, Mom phoned and remarked as an afterthought, "Oh, your father wants to die at home." At first I was afraid I'd misunderstood; then I was overjoyed. "We're going to be home together and care for Dad ourselves!" I thought. I couldn't wait to get to Texas. The hardest part—accepting that Dad was dying and making the decision where it would take place—was over.

Hunting season began. Dad was weak, in pain, and determined to go. Each weekend we bundled him up and prepared food he hardly ate, and his friends took him hunting. He sat in the open door of the cabin, a potbellied stove burning behind him. His rifle, almost too heavy to lift, sat on a table in front of him. He didn't shoot a deer, and it didn't matter. He was living: enjoying the silence of the country and the companionship of his friends, and forgetting, for a time, that he was dying.

When Dad walked out the door, we put him in God's hands and didn't worry about him...well, we worried just a little. His weekends away gave Mom and me time to take care of ourselves so we'd have the energy to care for him. I didn't have to wait up to make sure he remembered the 11:00 p.m. pain pills. Mom didn't have to wake up to help give the ones at 3:00 a.m., or worry about what to serve him for the next meal.

She dreaded figuring out what to feed him. There was little he could eat without gagging or throwing up, which was a physical problem that Mom took personally as a reflection of her ability to nourish. She was a gourmet cook, and sharing her love with food was no longer possible. It was a painful part of her process of letting go. During those weekends, she wasn't reminded at each meal that he was dying.

When Dad wasn't hunting, he sat in his reclining chair in the family room next to the patio doors. After a morning hug, he read the print off the newspapers as usual, played with the kids, worked on his taxpayer revolt, and directed the finishing of the cabin at the river that he and Mom had built with their own hands. Mom continued to keep their financial affairs in order. I remember Dad sitting in his chair, smiling and saying, "I feel so healthy I forget I have cancer." He was healthy in his heart.

Neighbors brought over banana pudding, casseroles, and roses, and prayed for our family. Dad's sister and her husband visited from New Jersey. Auntie Thelma, Mom's sister and our fairy godmother, called long distance twice a week. Friends phoned every day. It was difficult for the ones who visited to see Dad so weak. And it was as hard for them to express their feelings as it was for Dad to express his. Judy would come over after teaching to eat and play cards with Mom. She often felt frustrated about not knowing how to help Dad.

Ben, four, and Joshua, nine, brought a lot of joy to us all. As kids do, they went about playing as usual. As we shared their play, we'd forget about dying. They knew Gramps was dying, which meant he couldn't do all the things he used to do with them, and that he was going to die at home. Shining little Ben would come home from school and drop a drawing or lesson on Dad's lap for approval. Ben was learning to read, and they'd work together on letters and sounds.

For Joshua, coping with Gramps dying was more difficult. He'd recently left his father in Massachusetts, and now Gramps was going to leave too. Like his grandfather, he had difficulty expressing his feelings, so communicating was difficult. But he agreed with Ben, who said, "I like it better when Gramps is home." For his birthday, Josh was allowed to pick a dog from the pound. With Dad dying, we'd been concerned that a new dog would be just more complication; however, when he and Joshua enjoyed the dog so much, we wished we'd done it earlier!

At times, we all took it personally when Dad grouched because he was losing control of the few things he still felt he had command over. One night after Mom or Josh was in tears over one of Dad's grouches, I got angry. "Dad," I said, "everything that is flexible has to do with life, and everything that is rigid has to do with death. If people always have to play or do things your way, you may end up with no one to play with." It was an accomplishment for me to let him *see* me angry because he thought being angry was "losing control," and he'd never approved of it. Letting out my anger was healthy for me, and he understood.

Unlike Mary and John, Dad had pain that was difficult to control. The liver tumor expanded until it pressed against the nerves of the solar plexus. He was depressed because he constantly hurt physically. I guess he put up with the pain because he thought pain had to be part of dying. I told him, "You need your energy to live the time we have. There's no need to tough out the pain."

With the doctor's approval, we upped the Dilaudid from a usually potent 12 mg every four hours to even stronger dosages that would have been lethal for some. Before raising the dosage, we first tried other pain-relief techniques: breathing into the painful area, hot water bottles on his stomach and feet, hot cloths on his forehead. Sometimes we would just suffer through a painful period without raising the dosage. He wanted to keep the dosage down because he didn't like sleeping so much.

For nausea he took Compazine one hour before the Dilaudid; he also took Ritalin, a stimulant, twice a day to counteract the sedative action of Dilaudid. For general well-being, I gave him Bach flower remedies and massaged his feet once or twice daily, and of course gave him lots of love.

Although we appreciated having medical support available, we needed very little, except for information about and access to pain medication. We joined the St. Benedict Hospice Program so if we needed help, it could come to us. The hospice nurse visited three times, not because we needed her but because it was required by the program. It reassured Dad to question her about his symptoms. As for the rest of the family, it made me laugh with love to see us worry about not hurting the nurse's and social worker's feelings because we needed their help so little. If I hadn't had previous experience with dying, however, the program would have been invaluable.

Our chief outside supporter was Angie, the cancer research nurse from the VA, who soon became family. She became personally involved and worked with us as equals. She was the go-between for ourselves and Dr. Page. We phoned her with questions; she got answers, arranged prescriptions, and brought us medicine and supplies. This saved us running around when we had little extra energy.

Angie had me inject a needle into her arm to help me overcome the terror of shots I'd avoided facing with Mary. Because we'd traveled overseas a lot, I felt I'd spent half my childhood hiding under tables from people with needles. And now Dad might need methadone injections. One day Dad said, "Deborah, I need a shot," and I said, "Okay." Following the instructions in this book, I gave it to him. It was that simple. In my desire to help him, I forgot my fear. Love conquers fear.

Another day, at the time of the celebration over the return of the hostages from Iran, Dad was in pain and we'd done everything we knew how to do. I hated seeing him in pain, and I felt helpless and beaten. I went off alone and told God, "I've done my best and he's still in pain. He's in your hands. There must be something he has to learn from the pain."

When I stopped being Dad's protectress and accepted his pain (my pain), I felt at peace. Then a new idea came to me: I'd find some THC, the active ingredient in marijuana. It combats nausea and also reduces the amount of pain medication needed. He chose not to smoke marijuana but was willing to take socially and legally acceptable pills.

After we gave it to him, Dad became a beaming Buddha. He sat in his chair radiating sweetness and love. The THC appeared to open his awareness to his own nature; it also seemed to undermine his will, and will was all that was holding Dad in his body. By Sunday afternoon he was nearly dead. He sat in his chair and could not talk or move.

Suzy, Judy, Mom, and I gathered around him. With tears running down her face, Mom tried to wake him. She couldn't. This is it, we thought. Dad's dying now. We cried and told him we loved him. Mom remembered last rites. Should they be performed because Dad was raised a Catholic and still went to Mass twice a year? Suzy volunteered to find a priest and got on the phone. We were huddled around Dad when we heard her say, "Well, he's somewhat Catholic." We all burst out laughing. Tears of laughter mixed with tears of pain.

Neighbors appeared and told Dad they loved him. Someone put a cross beside him and a rosary in his hand. The priest came and went. Dr. Charlie appeared saying he'd just dropped in for a social visit. Actually, he'd driven fifteen miles because a neighbor had called and told him Dad was dying. "Yes," he agreed, Dad was dying. We decided to carry him to his bed.

Six of us lifted him in the air when Dad opened his eyes and said in a tone of surprise, "What's going on?" Laughing and crying we continued to carry him to his bed and tucked him in. Apparently, it wasn't his time yet.

Dad lived, actively, another two weeks. He continued to love swinging outside with us in the winter sun and playing with Joshua's new dog, Pizza. One of our last projects together was to paint Indian glyphs on a deerskin he'd tanned and stretched on a frame. The symbols he chose—three triangles, a man walking on water with an eagle coming out of his head, the sun, and two fish—revealed a man dying in peace.

Gradually he needed more attention. He used a cane to walk from the family room to the bathroom, ate almost nothing, and often seemed to drift away. He was so skinny that we put a foam pad on his chair and bed for comfort and to prevent bedsores. We dropped the schedule for pain medication and played it by ear. We'd discuss the amount he wanted and whether he wanted pills or shots, then arrange a schedule so Mom and I could sleep as much as possible.

Angie asked Dad if he was willing to be interviewed for a newspaper story on dying. Talking used a lot of energy but Dad said, "Fine, if it will help someone." The reporter asked how he'd decided to die at home. He said, "I knew Debby's friends who died, and their way sounded more like the way I wanted to go. I'd read her manuscript and heard about the hospice idea. I saw friends, fellow cancer patients, dying in the hospital...it seemed such an ignominious death."

The reporter asked Mom how she felt when Dad said he wanted to die at home. "If he was happier at home, we'd work it out," she replied in a quiet yet strong voice. "I couldn't have done this alone."

"What about joy and dying?" the reporter asked. Dad answered, "Well, at least you don't have any more problems!" He and Mom both said, "We don't know about joy, but we do feel peace."

"After you were diagnosed, how long was it before you could accept you were going to die?"

"Well, I was shocked. I felt angry and afraid and 'why me'—all those things you read about. Right after I heard I had cancer, I ran into a doctor who gave me hope. He told me it wasn't the end. His mother was a healthy eighty-six and had had cancer for years. I held on to 'It's not the end!'

"I'd like to tell people not to be afraid of dying. Dying gave me a chance to get rid of old sadness and feel peace. You can combine dying with your ordinary life. And doctors and nurses can help us get over the gap before we realize we can live while we're dying."

A few days after the interview, Dad said he didn't feel like walking to his chair. He stayed in bed except to go to the bathroom. Friends brought over foam wedges to prop up his legs and take pressure off his swollen ankles. Josh brought in his little TV.

That night we knew time was running out...and that it didn't exist. Mother and Dad rested together on their bed, leaning against each other. The beauty and peace in their faces spoke of the long journey they had shared together, and of the journey all people share. Love had made it worthwhile.

The next morning was surprisingly sunny and spring-like for February. I was happy padding around barefoot in jeans, shaving and bathing Dad. We were alone. Mom had secretly gone to check out funeral homes; Suzy was working on the first issue of the newspaper she was starting. The kids were at school. Dad and I talked.

He already knew I didn't believe death was the end, that we just leave a body that is no longer useful to us. We'd talked before about reincarnation and my memories of our being together in other times. This time we talked of preparations. I told him about spiritual teachings that suggest that when you feel yourself lifting out of your body, keep repeating "God" and follow the brightest light. Dad *heard me* and repeated, "Okay, remember to say 'God' and follow the light."

Our talk ended when Dr. Page arrived with Angie for a social visit. Dad was pleased Dr. Page cared enough to drive thirty-two miles round-trip on his lunch hour to visit. To him, that meant the doctor hadn't considered him just another number in the VA mill. Mom asked Dr. Page the old question, "How long?" He said, "Two days, two weeks!" I knew that was inaccurate.

We spent that evening around his bed. Dad played with Ben, rolling up a magazine telescope to watch him play hide-and-seek with himself. Josh said good-bye on his way out to Cub Scouts. Dad and I watched the world news to see if Poland was being invaded, as Mom worked on her *Saturday Review* double acrostic. Dad gave us instructions on the light fixtures at the cabin and on giving away his hunting guns. Suzy came in; Dad told her he loved her and repeated how much he loved us all. He considered phoning to ask Judy to come but decided it would worry her. "I'll *probably* be here in the morning."

Angie came in about nine p.m. out of a howling wind and rainstorm that came on the heels of a bright, sunny day. After she took his vital signs, she asked if she could stay over and sleep on the couch. While we sat around him visiting, Dad was looking at himself in the mirror across the room. Suddenly he stared and asked, "Do you see what I see?" I said I saw light all around him. He said he saw white light and rainbows, and when he saw the light, he knew he would die soon.

I asked again if he wanted me to call Judy, and he said yes. Judy came over and they joked together. "I love you, Judy," he told her. She said a teary good-bye. We kissed him goodnight, and he didn't speak again.

Mom and I were with Dad when he stopped breathing, a few hours past midnight on Wednesday, February 11, 1981. He was sixty-eight. Momma cried as she tucked the covers around him and said, "I love you, Daddy." I cried.

As I walked out into the dark, windy night and down the front yard path beside the stretcher with Dad's body, I remembered the words of Kahlil Gibran from *The Prophet:* "What is it to die but to stand naked in the wind and melt into the sun."

The ambulance waited as I said good-bye. "I love you, Papa. Stay with the brightest light."

I went back to the house and Mom and I crawled into her and Dad's bed. I heard Dad telling me, "If you hurt, let it out. Don't hold on until the pain cripples your will to live." I took time just now while writing this to cry again as I did that night. This time I lay on the floor, beating it with my arms, kicking, crying, and howling, to release the pain from my body. I heard a trapped animal freeing itself...myself.

That night Mom held me as I cried. Now I am alone with the beating of my heart—a heart opened wider after releasing the pain.

In the morning, I needed to clean. I washed clothes with fervor while Judy, Suzy, and Mom went to the funeral home. Dad wanted a military funeral with a GI's wooden box. This funeral home had no simple wooden coffins, so they chose a gray metal one. They arrived home saying, "It's a good thing you weren't there." (I knew I wouldn't deal well with the commercial aspect of burying people, which was precisely why I hadn't gone.) We joked about my idea of using an ice pick to punch holes in the box so earth could return to earth more quickly.

The next day was a blur. I planned the eulogy I would give at the funeral service. I'd asked Dad's permission and he'd said, "Okay, but keep it short." Suzy and I had the biggest fight we'd ever had. It grew out of unexpressed pain caused by neither of us feeling appreciated by the other. All my clothes were at the cabin, so I huffed off to buy something to wear. After Suzy's lecture on not always doing things my way, I thought maybe I should wear something conservative, not my usual style. Here I was, making a production over what to wear. Unbelievable!

At one point I was standing in total despair in a shop door at the mall, when a saleslady asked if she could help me. "I need a dress for my father's funeral." She said, "Oh yes, black," and I said, "Oh, no, white, purple, or peach!" I found a floaty peach dress that looked like "me" but chose a dark purple one so Mom and Dad's friends wouldn't be shocked. At home I told the story to Mom, who suggested, "Why don't you go back and get the peach one if it makes you happy?" I was repeating a lesson that was true for me: In the long run, doing what you want, instead of what you think you should, as long as you take responsibility for it, makes everyone happier.

I'm not sure if I steeled or centered myself to prepare for limousines, flower wreaths, all the funeral trappings the next morning. Last thing out the door, Mom, remembering our previous joke about earth returning to earth as quickly as possible, turned to me in mock seriousness and asked, "Have you got an ice pick?"

Joshua, who'd practiced reading the twenty-third Psalm the night before, backed out at the last minute. The part of me that was afraid to speak in public also wanted out. The rest of me wanted everyone to know Dad was alive and free.

With Dad's flag-draped coffin in front of me, I spoke shakily.

"My father is not dead. In this box in front of me lies only a shell. He's free and whole... Will you make today a day of joy and celebration as well as sadness?

"Dad said, 'I'm not happy about dying and I'm not afraid.' He believes we'll be together again.

"His cancer was a kind teacher. It gave him time to learn and to get his life in order...time to prepare for death. It taught him to give up control and surrender.

"Dad's death is a victory. He chose how he'd die. He chose to accept death, to accept life...Because he lives in our hearts, it's impossible to lose him."

A few weeks later, Mom, Ben, and I went back to the cemetery to put daisies on his grave. We all knew he wasn't there. I held Mom's hand and read:

Do not stand at my grave and weep
I am not there. I do not sleep.
I am a thousand winds that blow.
I am the diamond glints on snow.
I am the sunlight on ripened grain.
I am the gentle autumn's rain.
When you awaken in the morning's hush,
I am the swift uplifting rush
Of quiet birds in circled flight.
I am the soft stars that shine at night.
Do not stand at my grave and cry:
I am not there. I did not die.[2]

Ben and I sang "Zip-A-Dee Doo-Dah."

Aging is not for sissies.

—Bette Davis

2

MOM'S STORY

You can't prevent the birds of sadness from flying over your head,
But you can prevent them from making a nest in your hair.

—Chinese saying

Mom was sort of a female Will Rogers, quite ordinary and extraordinary. Remember Will Rogers saying, "I never met a man I didn't like"? Mom might have said the same. And I never met anyone who didn't like her. In simpler times, before women divided themselves between home and career, she totally devoted herself to her family's and friends' happiness and well-being.

A dear friend once said to me, "Your mother is the finest woman I've ever met." Unfortunately, he added, "Why aren't you more like her?"

Raised in the Ozzie and Harriet days of the 1950s, my sisters and I thought everybody's mom brought a tray with fresh strawberry shortcake, still warm from the oven, to their beds when they were sick. Or sewed doll clothes for you and all your girlfriends. Or had a special treat waiting when you got home from school, like a chocolate cupcake with your name on it, or a new organdy pinafore she'd sewn. We thought we were the best-dressed kids in school because she sewed our clothes. Living in a well-fortified ivory tower without knowing it, I thought store-bought clothes were for kids whose mothers were handicapped or didn't love them very much.

Although it seems unconscionably naive now, until freshman year in college I didn't know that not all families are happy. When I heard kids complaining that their parents sent them off to summer camp because they didn't want to be bothered with them, it was a revelation. In some ways, as children in a military family, we were quite isolated. We moved our loving cocoon from one location to another about every three years with little outside interference.

As the years passed, we—my sisters Judith and Suzanne and I—grew up, and life wasn't always so easy. Mom and Dad stood by us through broken hearts, broken backs, broken marriages, brain tumors, whatever—and we were loyal to them. Now, with Dad gone, we were totally devoted to Mom.

In the springtime, a year after Dad's cancer was diagnosed and the year before he died, Mom was diagnosed with Parkinson's disease. Perhaps the disease, latent in her body, was triggered by her grief over Dad's impending death.

For anyone, coming to terms with a chronic disease is a heroic journey. Mom did it with her customary grace: a blend of humor and stoicism. She didn't complain about having Parkinson's, losing the sight in one eye because a surgeon goofed, or shrinking a foot-and-a-half with osteoporosis and a hip fracture. Not one gripe! For her sake, I wish she had.

Whenever either of us had a new ache or pain, we'd look at each other and smile, and one of us would say, "Aging's not for sissies." Or she'd say, "You can't prevent the birds of sadness from…"

For what seemed like eons, but was actually twelve years, Parkinson's slowly and insidiously ate away at her body. We journeyed through increasingly distressing losses, from her handwriting diminishing in size—one of the first symptoms of Parkinson's—to her walk turning into a shuffle, to the constant shaking in her hands, to her finally being unable to walk, dress, or feed herself. For the last five years, she was virtually helpless, and we lifted her in the wheelchair to go to the bathroom or to go to town. She grieved quietly, as did her daughters, as her body's deterioration became stronger than her will.

During that time, an angel came into our lives. We called her Li'l Deb to distinguish her name from mine. Judy, Suzy, and I had all taken turns being Mom's primary caregiver. Now, she needed twenty-four-hour-a-day care, and we were in over our heads. Mom moved into a very fancy, yet wretched, nursing home in San Antonio. The saving grace was Li'l Deb, a beautiful young African-American woman who worked full-time at the nursing home and was also Mom's private sitter. You'd often catch them giggling together, joking, snuggling, or rubbing noses.

Considering her condition, Mom could have been strapped to a bed in the back ward; instead, she had a remarkable amount of fun. We bought Li'l Deb an old bomber Chevy station wagon with a hole in the exhaust pipe and a baseball cap emblazoned with the words *Driving Mrs. Duda.* Li'l Deb and Mom would tootle off on their adventures, like marching in the Martin Luther King Day parade. I still smile imagining my adorable eighty-two-year-old white mother in her wheelchair, wearing her baseball cap, among a sea of brown faces, smiling and waving to whomever—just glad to be outside under a blue sky. Even though her body no longer could, her spirit was standing up, making her statement for equality and justice.

As she shrank from a tall, robust woman to a tiny bird, her natural elegance shone through. On a number of occasions, as she was wheeled out to lunch at her favorite Italian restaurant, wearing oversized sunglasses, someone would say, "You look like Greta Garbo." Once she replied, "No, Greta Garbage." The name stuck in my heart.

Mom retained the twinkle in her eyes and a wry little smile, even when dealing with severe physical limitations and, later, bouts of dementia. She knew how to live in the moment.

She seemed to find life, with whatever limitations, precious. She found life meaningful in and of itself, simply because it is. She didn't ask life to perform, show off, or justify itself to her.

Mom's nursing home time was not easy for me, partially because I was still dealing with the guilt of reneging on my earlier promise to myself: "My mother will never go into a nursing home."

For the not quite two years she lived there, I regularly prayed for a way to bail her out. It seemed unfair that a woman who'd lived with so much love should die in a place she hated.

One day, I woke up telling myself the answer: We could rent a house near Judy (who lives in San Antonio), and Li'l Deb could live there with her three girls, and care for Mom. Mom would be in a real home again, with all the noisy, chaotic clutter of kids and animals underfoot. Instead of working fourteen hours a day at the nursing home, Li'l Deb could stay home and mother her girls. We would pay her salary and send her to nursing school so when Mom died she'd have a better life for her family. And in the mornings, when she went to nursing school, her mom could take care of my mom.

Excited, I called my sisters and Li'l Deb. Everyone agreed to the plan. And within a month, we did it. We heaved a communal sigh of relief. Everyone was happy again.

One Sunday near Christmas 1992, nearly a year after the move, I was happily decorating a tall noble pine with white-feathered doves and gold streamers in the living room of my house in Hawaii. I was thinking about Mom, because her Native American name, *Osoha*—her Bluebird den mother name—meant "tall pine." The phone rang. It was Li'l Deb. Her voice sounded strained.

"Something is different with your mom," she said. "She smells different."

"Do you think she's closer to dying?" I asked, because on my last visit, a month earlier, it had seemed she was approaching death.

"Yes," she replied.

"Okay," I said with surprising calm. "We need to know more or less how close so we can make plane reservations. Put her on the phone."

Since Dad's death and my writing *Coming Home,* talking honestly and openly about dying and death had become natural in our family. Being honest now with Mom was relatively easy.

"Momma, Li'l Deb says something has changed in your body and that you may be closer to dying. What do you think? What do you want us to do?"

Usually incoherent by now, with brief periods of lucidity, she couldn't answer in words. So Li'l Deb asked her questions and Mom replied by squeezing her hand. Deb reported, "She wants to go see a doctor."

"How strange," I thought. At Mom's request, we had avoided doctors as much as possible, and she had a living will. But, I reminded myself, "It's her life and she still makes the decisions."

Not having a family doctor, I said to Deb, "Call that doctor we saw at the nursing home. Make an appointment for tomorrow if you can, and put Mom back on the phone."

"Momma..." Teary, I paused. Only silence was big enough to hold a lifetime of love. My heart shared the gratitude that my mouth couldn't speak.

I prayed, "God, I hereby rescind my request to hold Mom in my arms when she dies. Please, whatever serves her highest good." And in a quiet knowingness, I accepted that my absence might be easier for her than my presence. Our emotional clinging to each other might slow down her leaving a miserable, deteriorated body. I felt peaceful.

"Mom," I said quietly, "for most of my life, the thought of someone I love dying at Christmas would have seemed horrible. But, if you need to go, I'd be happy to celebrate your birthday and Christmas together. I love you so much, Momma..."

In a muted, yet audible whisper, she said, "I love you."

❧

I telephoned Suzy and Judy and made airline reservations for the next night.

The night of the call, Li'l Deb, thinking Mom might die that very night, asked her, "Do you want me to stay in your room tonight?" Mom indicated, "No. You sleep in your own room."

The next day, Li'l Deb, who really wanted to stay close to Mom, said, "I don't have to go to school today. I could stay home with you."

Mom indicated, "No. You go to school."

When Deb got home from school that afternoon, she lifted my ninety-pound mother up in her arms, as we'd all done hundreds of times, and plopped her in the car. All the way to the doctor's office, she reported, Mom's usually closed eyes, which she often insisted she was just resting, were wide open. She looked at everything with intense interest.

At the doctor's office, Deb lifted Mom onto the white-papered examining table. Holding her wrist, the doctor looked worried. "I can't find her pulse...She won't live much longer."

Deb, taken aback at the imminence of what we had long been expecting, said, "But...will she die on the way home in the car?"

"Oh, no. Don't worry," the doctor nervously reassured Li'l Deb in a tone somewhere between consoling and patronizing. "She'll make it home just fine."

Mom just lay on the table smiling. At one point, she looked the doctor right in the eyes and grinned at him. Then, she looked at Li'l Deb, squeezed her hand, and grinned at her.

With a lilt in her voice, she said very clearly, "Bye." She took one deep breath and left her body.

Three minutes later, Li'l Deb phoned me.

"She's gone," she said simply.

Holding the phone in silence, looking out my window, I saw two monarch butterflies dancing around a pink flowering orchid tree. "There go Mom and Dad," I thought. "At last their love story has a happy ending."

Thinking of Mom, I smiled through my tears. "What an amazing woman! She planned where, when, and how she would die."

Mom was a very capable woman, an excellent organizer—a Leo with Capricorn rising, in case that has meaning to you. A month and a half earlier, she'd begun consciously refusing food and most liquids. She ate or drank only when pressured to by someone not yet ready for her to die. Mom knew, because I'd told her, that if she was tired of inhabiting her wretched little body, she could quit eating and drinking and she'd die of dehydration. She was courageous enough and/or had faith enough that death was not an end to literally starve herself to death.

I was certain that her surprising insistence on being taken to a doctor's office was not simply a whim. It was her thoughtful, tidy way of disposing of a body without disturbing and upsetting others. She knew from Dad's death that an unattended death at home requires a police visit, a painfully jarring experience for any family. She also knew we didn't have a doctor or nurse to sign the death certificate.

I imagined her smiling as she figured out, "The best place to dump a body is a doctor's office. Let them deal with it!" She wasn't fond of doctors. Perhaps grinning so intently at the doctor from his examining table was her way of saying, "Look here. I went to a lotta trouble to get here. If you think I'm taking this body home, guess again!"

❦

Now, years later, whenever I think of Mom and her death, or tell someone the story, I smile and feel totally at peace. What an incredible gift to give to our children: to die joyfully.

If one woman could smile and laugh at her death, then so can you and I. And without fear, the quality of life changes and death becomes a fresh breeze from God.

One joy scatters a hundred griefs.

—a Chinese proverb

3

MAKING THE DECISION TO DIE AT HOME

Everything can be taken from us but one thing: the last of the human freedoms—to choose one's attitude in any given set of circumstances, to choose one's own way.

—Viktor Frankl, *Man's Search for Meaning*
Survivor of Auschwitz and Dachau

When we can no longer control the circumstances of our lives, we can still choose our attitude about them. We can choose our attitude about dying. We can choose to see it as a tragedy, a teacher, an adventure, or simply as an experience to be lived. Our attitude will determine the nature of our experience. An optimist and a pessimist see the same world, only through different lenses. And as Norman Cousins said, "Pessimism is a waste of time. No one really knows enough to be a pessimist."[1]

When we choose to surrender to life, we are free; when we are free, we are in control. This paradox lies at the heart of our human existence.

To surrender and to be free we have to accept life as it *is* instead of holding on to how *we think it should be.* We can't change something we don't first accept. Surrender and acceptance are not to be confused with resignation and succumbing. Resignation and succumbing are *passive:* something just overpowered or overcame us and we had no choice but to give up. Resignation is self-pity and believing the illusion that we're powerless. Acceptance and surrender, on the other hand, are positive acts. "I choose to let go, to give up control and accept life as it is. And there will be things I can change and things I can't."

If we deny dying and death, we're prisoner to them. When we accept them, we're free and regain the power lost in resisting them. We let go of our resistance by letting go. It's easy to do and can be hard to get ready to do. The choice to let go must be made in the heart. A choice made only in the head, unsupported by the body, feelings, and soul, is unlikely to be carried out.

If we remember that choice of attitude, the ultimate freedom, is always available, we make a spacious place in which to experience dying. We can be free whether we are dying ourselves or sharing in the dying of someone we love. We can be free whether we die at home or in a hospital. Choosing our attitude is easier at home than in an atmosphere that isolates us from life.

As our Western culture emphasized control over nature, death became the uncontrollable enemy. We gave doctors the responsibility for combating this enemy. Death became increasingly a medical "problem" instead of a natural event. We gave away the responsibility for death (and life) to experts outside of ourselves: big institutions and big business. Until quite recently, life-sustaining technology said a good death is a hospital death and an unobstructed natural death is euthanasia. And people seemed to feel that because we invented machines, we have to use them. We became medical consumers with a mindset about life that was less about living and more about justifying our machinery.

Ivan Illich, in his scholarly and intriguing history of our attitudes and practices about death, *Medical Nemesis,* called death "the ultimate form of consumer resistance." Illich went on to say, "Today the man best protected against setting the stage for his own dying, is the sick person in critical condition. Society, acting through the medical system, decides when and after what indignities and mutilations he shall die."[2]

You may remember Karen Ann Quinlan, a young woman from New Jersey who brought to national attention the conflict between our technological capabilities and our human needs. In 1975, Karen became unconscious after mixing drugs and alcohol. A year later the courts upheld her *right to privacy* and gave her parents legal permission to refuse *extraordinary* treatment for her...even if that resulted in her death. Her respirator was removed, and Karen was moved to a nursing home.

Karen's parents decided to continue feeding her with tubes. One can only speculate on how being in the spotlight of national publicity and not having to pay for her care themselves affected the Quinlans' decision. Karen lived for ten years in a vegetative state with her expenses paid for by all us taxpayers. But the expense was perhaps well worth it, because she made us think together as Americans about the quality of life versus the quantity of life.

After she died in 1985, her mother, Julia Quinlan, said, "My daughter Karen's condition, like that of so many today, raised profoundly disturbing questions that do not lend themselves to easy answers or ideal situations. My hope and prayer is that medicine, technology and law will work together so that we will not become slaves to technology but rather, let technology with all its wonder enhance the worth, the dignity and the beauty of human life."[3] In many ways, Julia's prayer, the prayer about unnecessary human suffering, has been answered.

Now, in the early years of the twenty-first century, we've come a long way toward re-owning our humanity—ensuring kinder treatment for ourselves and our loved ones.

U.S. courts now uphold our *right* to privacy and to refuse *any* medical treatment we don't want—including feeding tubes and IVs—and our *right* to die with dignity. We now have legal documents—advance directives, health care proxies, durable powers of attorney, etc.—to protect us, to ensure that our wishes about our life and health care are carried out even if we can no longer express them ourselves.

In 1982, the Medicare Hospice Benefit was established. This legislation grew out of grassroots movements by hospices and holistic health practitioners, then considered to be on the fringes of medical treatment. Besides Cicely Saunders founding the first hospice (St Christopher's, in England), this legislation has had more influence on how dying Americans are treated and cared for than any other piece of legislation. Medicare was the first health care system in America to cover hospice-related services and led the way for Medicaid and private insurance companies to do the same.

Hospice and dying at home were ideas whose time had come. More and more courageous people were, and are, saying, "I don't want to go away to die. I want to die at home." Supported and stimulated by the financial backing of the U.S. government, the number of hospices has expanded from one in 1974 to over 4,850 in 2008.[4]

In 1986, the American Medical Association (AMA) finally got around to making an official policy statement that says it is ethically permissible for doctors to withhold all life-prolonging treatment, included artificial nutrition and hydration, from patients in irreversible coma and from others in terminal states.[5]

Palliative care and death and dying courses are now taught in universities and medical schools across the United States. Once again young doctors are recognizing the value of a family practice, personal care, and house calls.

We've come a long way. We're returning to dying at home: the old natural way of dying that most of the world doesn't question. However, because most Americans say they want to die at home and approximately 60 percent still die in hospitals or nursing homes,[6] we still have a long way to go.

We have a right to die with dignity. *Dignity* in the dictionary means "worthiness." To me it means doing things in our own way. In dying at home, we retain the ability to choose our own way, whether it be a little decision like what time we eat, or a big one like whether or not to enter a hospice program.

We have a right to die with respect—to see and to be seen. At home a person remains an individual rather than "The patient in room 204B."

Dying at home, we can influence the quality and quantity of our lives.

WHAT ARE THE ADVANTAGES OF DYING AT HOME?

(You may want to share this list with the dying person.)

1. Most dying people are happier at home than in a hospital.
2. The dying person can influence the quality and quantity of his or her own life.
3. Respect and dignity are maintained.
4. The dying person feels wanted.
5. You feel useful and needed.
6. The continued presence of love supports you both.
7. You both have more freedom and control. The dying person can tell you what he or she wants. (No one is awakened at 5:45 a.m. for temperature taking or another blood sample.)
8. You both can live more normally and fully.
9. The dying person can teach you something about living.
10. Home is more supportive of the shift from curing to making comfortable.

11. In a familiar and secure outer environment, both of you have more time for the inner preparations for death.
12. There is time and a place to express feelings of grief, anger, and love, so that accepting this death and death in general will be easier.
13. When physical death occurs, there's time to experience what's happened without the body being whisked away to make room for the next patient.
14. There's no travel wear-and-tear between home and hospital. (No worry about loved ones driving at night in bad weather.)
15. You both can see and create your own version of beauty.
16. Food at home can be fresher and more appetizing.
17. Living at home costs less.
18. Be it a slum or a palace, it's home!

I met a lovely ninety-two-year-old Spanish lady in the hospital who sat in a wheelchair hooked to tubes, chattering, mostly incoherently, about her bedspread at home, the curtains, and the good milk. It seemed to me she was still expressing what she wanted most: to be home. Home is a magic word.

WHEN IS IT NOT APPROPRIATE TO DIE AT HOME?

1. When the dying person doesn't want to.
2. When the family would be too upset to care for him or her.
3. When a hospital can provide services that improve the quality of the dying person's life.

4. When the dying person wants to be hooked into intravenous feedings (IVs), etc., and you can't afford a regular nurse.
5. When there is no one at home to care for the person and you can't afford to pay for someone.
6. It may not be appropriate if there are small children in the family, who also need care—not because it wouldn't be good for them to be present, but because you might not be able to manage it all. (If you can't get sufficient extra help at home, a residential hospice program may be a solution.)
7. If the dying person plans to donate organs for transplant, the death needs to take place in a hospital, because organs are transplanted soon after death.

MAKING THE DECISION

Sometimes it's very clear-cut. The person who is dying says, "I want to die at home" or just, "I want to go home." If this happens, the family can discuss among themselves whether or not this preference will work for everyone concerned. Your preferences, as well as the dying person's, need to be considered. The decision to come home must be a joint one. Only a family that wants someone to come home can give the care needed.

More often the situation is not so clear. The sick person still may hope to get better and may well do so. Or, someone may not know or want to know how sick she or he is, and feel anxious, afraid, and confused. Family and friends may feel the same. It's hard to feel clear about dying when we're getting a morass of conflicting reports from different parts of ourselves; the body, mind, feelings, and soul each report their own story or reality.

In the face of death, the rational mind is afraid because it can't understand or control what's happening. It *thinks* death is the end and fights it. The body's job is to stay alive. It *senses* that death means extinction and fights it. The *feelings* are confused because their work is to react to the other parts. The part that endures, the soul or consciousness, seems to make an arbitrary decision to leave, which instigates death, and then can't understand why body, mind, and feelings resist and make such a fuss.

No wonder we feel confused by dying and death and often wonder what the heck is going on.

Only the heart is not confused. It *knows* the larger plan. It intuitively knows the whole. It *loves* each part and understands the sacredness of each. It *sees* the truth: life without the lens of fear. When we accept all the parts of ourselves and surrender, the heart opens wide, the conflicting reports end, and we can live fully with dying. Mind, body, feelings and soul are aligned so we can make decisions based on all our needs.

If this feels like a tall order for you now, keep in mind it can take a long time to accept ourselves fully. We can practice by surrendering for brief moments at a time.

Give loving support and information to help everyone involved make the best decision possible at this time. Include in the information what the patient wants to do, what you want to do, finances, your own state of health, child care, and the availability of help. To avoid total exhaustion, I recommend there be at least two people at home to take turns supporting the dying person. In the following section on financial considerations, and in chapter 4, you'll find more information to help with the decision.

You'll probably want to discuss your choices with your doctor and/or a hospice doctor. Remember, a doctor in this circumstance is a provider of information, not a decision maker. Many doctors are accustomed to recommending the hospital for very sick people. If a hospital is recommended, ask how it can serve the dying person.

The availability of a hospice in your area may be an important factor in your decision about whether or not a home dying and death is appropriate for your family. Hospice is a service to help the dying and their families at home. Their services include

- physicians;
- nursing care;
- physical, occupational, and speech therapy;
- medical social services;
- home health aides;
- homemakers;
- medical supplies, including drugs and medical appliances;
- counseling, including dietary and bereavement;
- short-term inpatient care for respite care, pain control, and symptom management.

If the dying person is eligible for Medicare, call your local hospice and ask if they're Medicare approved. Most insurance policies cover hospice care, as does Medicaid in most states.

Sometimes people are afraid to enter a hospice program because they think it means they are "giving up." To the contrary, it means you are choosing quality of life. To enter a hospice program, your doctor and the hospice medical director have to certify that you have six months or less to live. But, the decision to enter a hospice need not be permanent. You can leave the program at any time, for whatever reason. For example, your loved one's cancer may go into remission, or another healing miracle may happen, and you no longer need hospice services. You can always leave the program and enter it again if you need it.

As mentioned before, you may find it surprising to know that in 2009 the National Hospice and Palliative Care Organization reported, based on their study of terminally ill patients using hospice versus those in a hospital or nursing home, that the mean survival period was twenty-nine days longer for hospice users.[7]

Whatever decision you make, remember it need not be permanent. If a person is at home and you still have doubts or it's not working out, a hospital or nursing home is always available. Returning someone can be emotionally difficult for all concerned, and sometimes it's necessary. Respect your feelings. You are just as valuable as the dying person.

Examine your motives carefully before bringing or keeping someone home. If guilt is the motive ("If I were a good person, I'd bring her home" or "I *should* bring him home"), you might not have the energy to keep going. Love sustains us; guilt drains us.

Resentment begins with feeling or thinking someone *should* do or be something they aren't. "He *should* be cooperative" or "She *should* feel grateful." Keep in mind that people bring the same characteristics to dying that they do to living. A person with a difficult or demanding personality generally dies true to character. Although the process of dying may transform a personality, it would be foolish to expect it. Do you want to care for the person just as she or he is now? If you do, you will generally be able to meet the challenges. There will be challenges, and each is an opportunity for growth.

Pain management is one of the great fears of the dying and their families. In most cases pain can be alleviated just as well at home as in the hospital. Hospice and palliative care doctors are medical pain management pros. In my experience, dying people living at home have less pain than those in a hospital. Love is a very effective stress and pain reducer. If the dying person cannot take pills or liquids, a transdermal patch may be effective, or a nurse can give injections or teach you to give them. With a nurse's help, even IVs can come home. Pain control isn't something to fear, just something to do.

Another fear of a dying person is, "What will happen to my family?" When he or she sees you at home coping with and competently handling this terminal illness, the fear will be alleviated. At home there's time for making the appropriate arrangements.

Dying people also fear being a burden. Reassure them they're not and that their dying process is part of the whole family's life. For example, when I suggested coming home while Dad was dying, Mom said, "But you've got to get on with your life, Deborah." My response was, "What happens in my family is part of my life." You might say to someone who wants to be at home but who fears being a burden, "Allowing ourselves to receive love and caring is just as important as giving them. Please let us return some of the love you've given to us by allowing us to care for you at home." Or to a really stubborn person, "Are you going to give the pleasure and privilege of caring for you to your family or to strangers?"

Dying people, as well as a lot of the rest of us, fear loneliness and being deserted. In Malcolm Muggeridge's *Something Beautiful for God,* he quotes Mother Teresa: "I have come more and more to realize that it is being unwanted that is the worst disease that any human being can ever experience... For all kinds of diseases there are medicines and cures. But for being unwanted, except there are willing hands to serve and there's a loving heart to love, I don't think this terrible disease can ever be cured."[8]

Bringing dying people home reassures them they're wanted and won't be deserted. And we may have to reassure them many times. Being at home also alleviates loneliness.

Dying people fear losing control over their lives. In the hospital, the staff takes over and largely dictates what the patient can and must do, when you can see them, etc. The result is, you and the dying person don't have time to adjust gradually to the loss of control. At home, on the other hand, you can take a few steps at a time toward giving up control, which makes dying easier.

The feeling of being totally wrenched by an unnatural catastrophe, common in sudden deaths and many hospital deaths, is less likely to occur at home. When you care for someone at home, you have the satisfaction of knowing that you're doing all you can do. If the thought comes up afterward, "Maybe I could have done more," you're likely to let go of it much more quickly than if you'd been isolated from a loved one. After caring for someone who dies at home, most people report feeling peace as well as loss—a feeling of appropriateness and completion and a greater openness to the new life ahead. Mom said, "I feel good because Dad was so happy to be at home and die the way he wanted to."

Sometimes the dying person is medically termed "unconscious" but has earlier expressed a desire to be home or has signed an advance directive, a living will. This is a document we can sign any time in our adult lives instructing doctors to withhold or withdraw extraordinary life-sustaining procedures during a terminal illness. (See the section in chapter 11 "Advance Directives, Living Wills, and Health Care Proxies.")

Patients whose level of consciousness is uncertain may still let us know what they want. You can ask, for example, "Do you want to go home? Squeeze my hand for yes; blink for no." Use whatever signal you can invent using the abilities the person still has available.

Few people realize we have the legal right to leave a hospital whenever we please, with or without a doctor's approval. A family has the legal right to make a decision for a person who is "incompetent," not able to make or express his or her own decisions. Under these circumstances, the next of kin can take responsibility for checking the patient out of the hospital. You may have to sign a form stating that the patient is leaving the hospital against medical advice (AMA). Attending physicians most frequently just drop a case if they don't agree, but they can resort to legal proceedings if they feel it's not in the best interest of the patient to leave. This is uncommon because all states now have advance directive laws that legally protect our right to refuse treatment. In 1992, the American Hospital Association drew up a patients' bill of rights that also affirms that right. Check with your insurance provider to make sure they will cover your medical expenses if a patient leaves the hospital against medical advice.

What is in the *best interest* of a person who hasn't expressed his or her wishes in an advance directive and now can't express them? This is a difficult one. What is the quality of life of someone in a coma, sustained by tubes, with little chance of functioning alone again? What is in the best interest of a patient who had expressed a desire to go home?

Here, some profound thinking is necessary about the quality of life versus the quantity. In a hospital a person may be kept alive longer, but in what condition? What is the difference between a coma in which consciousness lifts out of the body to allow the body to restore itself, and a coma in which consciousness leaves to prepare the body for death? When does physical survival cease to be a desirable goal? Each case is different. I believe answers come from an inner or higher source that we can reach through prayer and meditation.

Keeping in mind the considerations mentioned that are relevant for you, why not gather as a family to discuss the idea of bringing or keeping someone at home? Then perhaps each individual separately can pray, meditate, think, and feel about the choices. At least sleep overnight before coming together again to share your preferences. If your decision is "home," affirm it together, recognizing that you may still have doubts and that together you'll do your best. Not everyone has to do everything; one person may want to physically care for the person, another may prefer caring for the children. Remember you're a team. If the decision is "hospital," be assured that the decision you make is the appropriate one at the time.

The gathering could be a time to make an agreement that may save needless suffering later. It can happen that a medicine or something else we give the dying person speeds up the process of leaving the body. We cannot know the effects on each individual of all foods, medicine, and treatments. Affirm together that if a dying person dies as a result of something you administer with the best intentions, there's no need for guilt or blame. God or the mysterious and subtle workings of the universe simply used you to help that person out of their body at that time. You are aligned with your purpose: allowing someone to die at home with love around them. If this responsibility is too heavy for you to handle, a nurse may be hired.

In this gathering of family and friends, you may want to express your love and support for each other. Sharing loving energy will strengthen each of you. Whoever needs to share in this dying is who needs to be present for it.

Once you've made the decision for home, keep in mind that your focus must shift from *curing* to *making comfortable.* Now, do everything possible for comfort rather than to prolong life, as long as the dying person is in agreement. A dying person may want to prolong life for some reason: seeing a son or daughter graduate from school, a grandchild born, etc. People have a right to change their decisions.

FINANACIAL CONSIDERATIONS

Finances will probably be a factor in your decision. It's generally less expensive to die at home. John and Mary, for example, had few additional expenses; my father had none. For Mom, renting a house and paying for a caregiver were less expensive than the nursing home.

As I mentioned earlier, to keep or bring a dying person home, there must be at least two people to care for him or her. If you're working, can you arrange leave from work? Can you afford to? Can you work part-time? A 1993 law, the Federal Family and Medical Leave Act, guarantees up to twelve weeks a year of unpaid leave for caring for a sick child, spouse, or parent. This law covers all U.S. government and state employees and employees of companies with fifty or more employees. (If we lived in Denmark or Sweden, the leave would be paid for!)

Some employers may allow sick and vacation leave to be used during this time to mitigate the financial burden. Some institutions even have sick leave pools, whereby you can petition to be granted extra paid leave out of a pool of other workers' donated extra or unused leave.

Hospice services are covered by Medicare, Medicaid, Veteran's Administration, private insurance plans, HMOs, etc. Do you have hospice coverage or coverage for home-care services such as nurse visits and medicine? If you don't have insurance coverage, can you afford a nurse or doctor if they're needed?

If there's a hospice in your area and you don't have insurance, call them anyway. Often their fees are on a sliding scale dependent upon your income. Many, but not all, have special funds that enable them to take care of a dying person who can't pay. Hospice benefits do not cover room and board charges in hospitals or nursing homes.

Medicare hospice coverage does not pay for treatment other than for pain relief and symptom management for a terminal illness. You pay no more than five dollars for each prescription drug and other products for pain relief and symptom control. For respite care, which is a short hospital or nursing home visit for the dying person to give the family a needed rest, you pay 5 percent of Medicare's cost.

Even if there's no hospice in your area, Medicare and Medicaid cover home care if there's a medically established need for "skilled service." The service must be given by a certified home health care agency under a doctor's direction. Both programs require an "assessment visit" by a registered nurse.

Now, let's look at private insurance policies. If you have one, check to see if it covers hospice care; most do. If not, what coverage is provided for home visits by a doctor or nurse? Insurance often covers 80 percent of the cost after a $100 deductible or 100 percent after $1,000. What are the limitations on home-care services? Nearly all policies specify a maximum number of visits covered. If the policy is written in Greek, call an insurance agent and ask him or her to explain the benefits to you.

Keep in mind that insurance companies are run by people. It's possible to negotiate with them. If your insurance doesn't cover home care, consider asking your agent for help. You might say, "My policy with you doesn't cover home care, but it does cover hospital care. If you will finance home care, it will save you a lot of money!" Sometimes you can work out an arrangement.

If there's no hospice and you don't have insurance, check the availability and cost of doctor and nurses' visits. Look under "nurses" in the yellow pages. Getting prices by phone may be difficult, but you can often arrange a free nursing assessment visit in your home.

Nurses are categorized according to education and skills. For example, generally only a registered nurse (RN) can start IVs and give injections. A licensed vocational nurse (LVN) provides general nursing skills such as monitoring vital signs and changing dressings. Home health aides do bathing, personal care, housekeeping, and running errands. Nursing costs vary, so shop for the qualifications you need at the best prices. The more training a nurse has, the more you pay, so don't hire an RN to help bathe someone, unless you enjoy giving money away.

Visiting nurse associations (VNA) are nonprofit nursing organizations. Their fee scale and services are similar to profit-making nursing agencies. Many of them receive funds from United Way and provide sliding fee services. Most nursing agencies divide their services into two categories: private duty nursing visits and home health aide visits. Let them know what you need. You might call your county government to check if they have a home health care service or a public health nurse who makes home visits without charge.

You can also find a nurse through referrals or a newspaper ad. You may find a wonderful one and pay less. You will have to trust your own judgment because you won't have outside assurance about reliability and skill.

Talk with the nurse or nursing agency about your needs and resources. Unless you're working and need full-time support, a nurse can train the family in ordinary nursing skills. You need to call only in the event of unusual challenges. In many cases only a few short visits are needed. Mary had about six, and Dad had three. The price of doctors' visits also varies, so call and ask. Again, let them know your needs and resources. You may not need a visit by a doctor or nurse. We didn't with Dad, although some visited because they wanted to.

For further information on financial help, check the following sections in chapter 4: "City, County, and State Services," "Social Security," and "Veterans Administration."

Serving humanity is recognizing
our common divinity.

—Phoebe Hummel

4

SOURCES OF HELP

Called or not called, God is always here.

—Carl Jung

In one morning on the telephone, you can find out a lot that will help you make your decision or, if you've already made it, get you started finding help if you need it. Here are some resources that may be of help. You'll probably find others. New alternatives and possibilities spring up every day.

If someone says, "No, we can't help," ask if they know who can. Keep a list of the useful numbers by your phone. When Mary was dying, we had a bowl on the kitchen table where we put all those notes we wrote about possible help. Share with the dying person what you find out unless it's clearly inappropriate.

Whether you need a little or a lot of help, you'll probably feel more comfortable knowing where to get it if you need it in a hurry.

FAMILY AND FRIENDS

Family and friends may be your biggest help. Let them know that this person they're close to is sick and probably dying, that you're planning a home death, and ask if they're willing and able to help. You do them a favor by offering the opportunity to give of themselves and to face their own fears about dying.

People basically love to help and to feel needed. Your request might give someone who at the moment is experiencing life as meaningless an opportunity to find meaning. There's no need to think you're imposing by asking; everyone is free to say no. Present a clear opportunity to which yes or no are equally valid responses. For example, "John is dying at home and we need help running errands, cooking meals, caring for him, etc. Is this a time in your life when you can help?" Let them know you're aware that there are times when it's not possible, and that's fine. It may happen that some of your inner circle of friends may not be ready to face their own feelings about death and may move to the outer circle. People you hardly knew before may move to the inner circle.

What about forming a neighborhood co-op to care for the sick and dying—a caring network? It would take a fair amount of courage for the first person to reach out, but it could totally change our feeling of separateness—living isolated lives in city apartments and suburban homes. Starting a caring co-op might take just one phone call to those neighbors you don't know or one meeting at your house to ask for help. It might be organized around your husband, wife, or child, then spread to include everyone in the neighborhood. Ms. Johnson can come over for an hour and sit with John. Julie can come over after school and tidy up. Mr. Smith can mow the lawn. Mrs. Martinez can't come over but can bake a casserole. The Dudas could have the kids over to play. Mr. and Mrs. Levy can come over and sit with John and watch TV while you get away to the movies. Imagine what would happen to a neighborhood or an apartment house with everyone cooperating, feeling needed, having a sense of purpose, and learning to love each other. What a joyful prospect.

MEDICAL AND HOME CARE HELP

Hospices

A hospice is a public agency or private organization that helps families care for a dying loved one at home. Some of the most loving, compassionate people you will ever meet are hospice staff members and volunteers. If there's a hospice in your community, they can give most of the help you'll need.

Hospice is a relatively new word in American health care. It comes from the Latin word *hospes* which meant someone who hosted a guest or stranger. Later, in the Middle Ages at the time of the holy pilgrimages, *hospice* meant a "way station," a place for tired, sick pilgrims to receive care. *Hospes* is the root word for "hospitality" and "hospital."

The hospice idea was revived by a courageous English woman, Dr. Cicely Saunders, who was unhappy about the way her dying patients were treated in hospitals. To her, hospice meant a way station between this world and the next. The hospice she began in 1967 in London, St Christopher's Hospice, generated enthusiasm all over the world for better care of the dying. Today there are about 200 hospices in England and, as I said before, over 4,850 in the United States.

The main concern of a hospice program is to help patients live until they die and for their families to live as fully as they can while their loved one is dying...and to go on living afterward. A team of caregivers, including a doctor, nurse, social worker, counselor, chaplain, and volunteers, becomes personally involved with you and the dying person, to the degree that you choose.

All hospices emphasize care at home. If you and a dying family member have chosen dying at home, you may feel more secure knowing a hospice nurse is on call 24/7, and able to visit you at home when necessary. If dying at home is not appropriate, you might check with your local hospice anyway. About 20 percent have their own facility with a home-like supportive atmosphere, and some hospitals have a hospice unit in which hospice-like care is given.

Hospices generally accept only patients who have been certified by their doctors as having a life expectancy of six months or less. Their emphasis is on alleviating symptoms rather than curing disease. Sophisticated pain control techniques allow most patients to live their remaining time pain free and alert.

Hospices also provide respite care and bereavement support.

To locate a hospice in your area, check the telephone book under "hospice," call your hospital, or call the National Hospice and Palliative Care Organization at 1–800–658–8898.

Visiting Nurses

If you don't have a hospice in your area, you can usually still manage caring for someone at home. You will have to shop around to find the services you need, like nursing assistance. If you have private insurance, check your policy. What coverage does it provide for nursing care at home?

To locate a nurse, look in the yellow pages under "nurses" or "nursing services." Call the agencies in your area and compare costs and qualifications. Don't forget to check if your county has a public health nurse who makes free home visits.

A visiting nurse can teach you basic nursing skills that relate to providing comfort, moving a patient, changing sheets, bathing, and exercising. They can show you how to give non-intravenous injections and can advise on feeding problems, enemas, and other patient needs. They can answer many patient's questions and recognize when a doctor is needed.

Home Health Care Aides

Another important kind of assistance comes from home health care aides. Their services may include personal care, homemaker services, transportation and escort, and companionship. They can help the patient to eat, dress, bathe, and make beds, tidy up rooms, and help the patient to get in and out of bed or take walks. Their training, supervision, and cost vary, so check around.

There's not yet a national certification program, although to work in a Medicare-funded program, home health care aides must have passed a qualifying exam. Many home health care aides are state certified after completing a training program.

To find an aide, call a medical social worker at a hospital to recommend an agency. Look in the yellow pages under "homemaker-home health aide services," "visiting nurse associations," "family service agencies," or "social service agencies."

Eldercare

The Administration on Aging (AoA), part of the U.S. Department of Health and Human Services, was created to help older people live independently. Their web site, www.aoa.gov, includes links to state and local agencies on aging, and community organizations that serve older adults and caregivers.

Eldercare Locator, part of the AoA, can help you locate services in your community from Meals on Wheels to home health aides. Call 1–800–677–1116 from 9:00 a.m. to 9:00 p.m. or go to the web site, www.eldercare.gov. You type in the service you want and your zip code, and it gives you names and contact information for appropriate agencies in your area.

Hospitals

A hospital is always available if you need one. You can use one for particular services, even though the intention is to die at home. If your patient does have to go into a hospital for some treatment that will improve the quality of life, I recommend not leaving him or her there alone. Nurses, no matter how excellent, don't have time to attend to all the emotional and physical needs of their patients. If you do have to leave someone, don't feel guilty. They'll manage, and perhaps they have something to learn on their own.

Even if you don't use a hospital, you can call the hospital's director of nursing services for information about other services in your community.

Social Security

Besides Social Security retirement benefits, Social Security administers five programs that may be useful to you and the dying person: Medicare, disability insurance, dependent benefits, survivors' benefits, and supplemental security income. They also determine eligibility for Medicaid in some cases.

The problem we encountered with Social Security in Mary's case was that their help didn't arrive before she died. With luck, you'll have more time, and the application processing will be complete in time to be fully useful. Ask about presumptive eligibility, which is designed to speed up the process.

Retirement Benefits. If you're sixty-two and have paid enough into Social Security, you're eligible for monthly payments.

Medicare. If you're sixty-five and have paid enough into Social Security, you're eligible for Medicare. Medicare is a health insurance program similar to private health insurance. There's generally a deductible, and the policy pays a certain percentage over the deductible.

Medicare will pay for hospice care provided by a certified hospice, or occasional part-time skilled nursing services, home health aides, or medical social worker services, and for some medical supplies and appliances prescribed by a doctor and furnished by a certified home health care agency.

If you already have Medicare, find a hospice or home nursing service that's certified by them. For more information, call your local Social Security office and ask them to send you the handbook "Medicare & You."

Disability Insurance Benefits. Regardless of age, if you're totally disabled and a doctor says you can't work for twelve months, or your disability is likely to result in death, you can receive monthly payments *if* you've paid enough into the system. Social Security requests reports from your doctor and determines if you're disabled.

You have to work under Social Security for five out of ten years before you were disabled to be eligible. There's a five-month waiting period when no disability benefits are paid. Payments start on the sixth month from the beginning of the disability.

Dependent Benefits. A spouse who is sixty-two or older, people who have a disabled child in their care, or children under sixteen may be eligible for payments.

Survivors' Benefits. When a wage earner who has paid into Social Security dies, his or her survivors are eligible for the following:

- A lump sum burial payment up to $255 payable only to a surviving spouse or a child entitled to monthly benefits.
- Monthly payments to a widow or widower sixty years old or, if disabled, at fifty years; a divorced widow or widower married ten years; a minor child to sixteen years; dependent parents; a widow or widower caring for a child under sixteen or a disabled child (eligible for life if applied for before age twenty-two).

Supplemental Security Income. This program is based on need, not on your having paid anything to the government. If you're sixty-five, blind, or totally disabled, the government will supplement your monthly income. The amount goes up every January. Your resources must not exceed a certain level, and they don't count the value of a house, the land it's on, nor a car. Most states supplement supplemental security income and pay higher amounts.

Medicaid

Medicaid is a state-administered health program for people with low income based on need. Medicaid, unlike Medicare, pays nearly all medical expenses. There's no deductible. In some states you apply for Medicaid at your local welfare office, in others at a Social Security administration office.

If you have questions about Medicaid, call your state welfare department or department of human resources.

For questions about other federal programs, call your nearest Social Security administration office or 1–800–772–1213. Much of your business can be completed by phone. If you need to see them in person, ask which documents to bring so you don't waste a trip. If you're applying by phone, make a note of the date, whom you spoke with, and the subject of the conversation in case you have to call again. To avoid a long wait, don't go on Monday, which is usually their busiest day.

Veterans Administration

In your area there is a veterans' service bureau or agency. [1]

Any person who served in the U.S. Armed Forces with at least ninety days of wartime service and an honorable general discharge, and who's over sixty-five or totally and permanently disabled, is eligible for a pension. In 2009, a single vet could receive up to $490 per month; a married vet could receive $642 plus $84 a month for each dependent child. All your income is counted against the $490—they pay you the difference. And how many people can live on that? This is a shame.

Depending on their income, a widow or dependent children of a vet are eligible for a pension and educational benefits. If the death is "service-connected" (for example, the vet dies of an old wound, illness, or condition acquired while in the service), there are additional benefits.

Eligible vets who need help caring for themselves can receive an "aid-in-attendance allowance" of up to $937 if married or $785 if single. "Housebound" vets unable to leave home but who do not need other help are eligible for up to $600 a month if single and $752 if married.

If a vet has to go to a private hospital in an emergency, the receiving physician must call a VA hospital within seventy-two hours. If he or she is eligible, the VA will transfer the vet to a free VA hospital or pick up the tab if the vet is too ill to be transferred. When a vet dies in a VA hospital or while being transferred to one, the VA will pay to transport the body to the hometown or place of burial.

A vet, his widow, and any number of unmarried children under eighteen can receive a plot and headstone free of charge in a national cemetery. If a vet who is receiving a pension or compensation for service-connected disabilities is buried in a private cemetery, the VA will pay up to $500 for burial and up to $300 for plot and interment. If the death is "service connected," there's a burial allowance up to $2,000. The VA will also furnish headstones and a burial flag. Funeral directors have the applications for burial benefits and will complete them for you, or you may apply at the nearest VA office.

The VA doesn't chase you around the country to give you money. You have to apply. They have other benefits not mentioned here, and their laws and payments change often, so check with the VA. Visit their web site at www.va.gov, or call 1-800-827-1000 to get the number of your regional office.

LEGAL HELP

Legal Aid Services

These are government-funded, nonprofit services that can help with any type of legal problem, including land transfers, wills, and estate planning. There are certain income qualifications for receiving these no-cost services.

To find a legal aid service, look in the yellow pages under "attorney" or "social service organizations." If you can't find one there, call the county courthouse, bar association, or a lawyer referral service.

State Boards of Health, Medical Examiners, County Coroners

At some point you'll need to know about the laws in your area regarding death at home and burial. This will enable you to plan a simple, dignified funeral that meets your needs and desires, as well as the legal requirements.

Look in the white pages under the name of your state, county, or city for the local "board of health," "medical examiner," or "coroner," or call your hospital or county courthouse and ask who to call.

MEDICAL SUPPLIES

Rental Services

Many types of medical supplies are covered by Medicare and by private insurance policies. Check your policies to find out what supplies are covered.

Hospices provide most of the supplies you'll need. If you're not working with a hospice, you can rent supplies such as hospital beds, wheelchairs, and commodes. Check if they are available free of charge from nonprofit organizations. If not, rent by the month; the rates are lower. Look in the yellow pages under "medical supplies—rental" or "rental services."

Medical supply companies or pharmacies near a hospital specialize in selling supplies needed by patients at home. You can also order all types of medical supplies online.

American Cancer Society

Local chapters of the American Cancer Society want to be as helpful as possible to their communities. Different chapters provide different services or supplies, such as wheelchairs, dressings, or disposable pads for incontinent patients. They often provide free transportation to and from treatment. Some have wigs available for women who've lost their hair due to chemotherapy.

COUNSELORS

Counselors are people specially trained to help us with our feelings. If this dying process brings up feelings that you have difficulty dealing with, consider getting outside help, such as a therapist, psychologist, or social worker. It's a sign of courage, not cowardice, to seek help from a professional if problems seem beyond your capacity to handle at this particular time.

Hospices have counselors, or you may already know people in your community who specialize in helping people face emotional challenges. Finding someone who is relatively clear about his or her own feelings about death will be most helpful. Call a hospice for recommendations. Check with a county mental health association, a community mental health clinic, or a college. If you live in a city, look for a council of social agencies or a branch of the Family Services Association. For a child, you might check first with the school guidance counselor.

SPIRITUAL SUPPORT

Churches and Synagogues

Your priest, minister, or rabbi will want to visit and share their compassion and services with you and the dying person. Obviously the richness of your spiritual and religious life will support you as you face dying.

Calling a clergyperson or rabbi is clearly the choice of the dying person. It would be disrespectful for the family or clergy not to accept a dying person as he or she is by attempting a last-minute conversion.

A priest can be called at any time to perform the anointing of the sick, a celebration of God's healing sacrament. Previously called "last rites," it is now given at any time to the sick, elderly, or dying.

There are no deathbed sacraments in Judaism, although there is a tradition of *vidui,* a statement of confession as death approaches. This may be the recital of the Shema as an affirmation of faith or the traditional prayer for the dying. From ancient times, Jewish tradition has prescribed a mourning ritual which is compatible with modern understandings about the grieving process.

EMERGENCY SUPPORT

Fire Departments and Emergency Medical Services (EMS)

In some places the fire department and EMS are in the same department; in others, not.

Fire departments are close to my heart because they seem to work on the principle of brotherly/sisterly love. Without their help, we couldn't have gotten Mary out of that second-story apartment! Many fire chiefs have told me to tell you, "If you need help, call us. We'll try to help you or find someone who can." How's that for reassuring?

Both EMS and fire department staffs are trained to solve unusual problems. For example, if you're alone—no neighbors are home—and the person you're caring for falls out of bed and you need help to get them back in, they can assist you. EMS specializes in out-of-hospital acute care and transporting people to a hospital, and they're available for any lifesaving activity.

For emergency help, call 911. It connects you to a central emergency information service that will connect you to EMS or the fire department. If you speak with EMS, make it clear that you're supporting a home dying and don't want the person taken to the hospital, if that's true. If your area doesn't use 911, call the fire department. If you are working with a hospice, call them instead of 911. Calling 911 may terminate hospice insurance benefits because it's considered a lifesaving measure and therefore doesn't meet the hospice mandate to provide comfort.

Ambulances

In case you have to move someone from one place to another who can't be moved by car, van, or pickup, find out ahead of time about ambulance services and costs. They generally require cash upon delivering the person. So, be prepared.

He who binds to himself a joy
Does the winged life destroy;
But he who kisses the joy as it flies,
Lives in eternity's sunrise.

—William Blake
Notebook

5

GETTING ON WITH IT: PREPARATIONS AND HOMECOMING

Being deeply loved by someone gives you strength,
while loving someone deeply gives you courage.

—Lao-Tse
Chinese Taoist philosopher

Know that you are not alone. Every heart in the world is part of every other heart. Even if there is no friend or family beside you, you are not alone. The energy that created and encompasses us is with us as we bring someone home to live until they die.

Strength beyond what you imagine is yours. Love protects and surrounds you as you meet each task of the day.

The everyday limits of time and space can be transformed into a sense of connectedness with all people if you expand the frame around your experience with dying. If you're feeling alone—as if everything is closing in or you just walked into a wall—close your eyes and imagine yourself as part of a huge family that's experiencing the same things you are, even in the same moment. Think of the people before you who have experienced dying—family, friends, people you don't even know—and all of us who will experience it in the not-so-distant future.

Each heart in the world standing beside someone they love who is dying is connected with ever other heart. Approximately 200,000 members of our family die each day on our planet—about 6,700 in the United States.[1]

If you feel your heart is breaking, feel it breaking open. Hearts don't break closed. People close them. The courage or peace you may find in your Self is shared with us all.

Whenever you're troubled or don't know what to do next, ask for guidance from the quietest, deepest place you can find in yourself...and listen for the answer. Sooner or later you'll hear it. It will come with quiet reassurance. Trust what you hear. Your Self knows more than all those experts out there. Embrace your sadness and fear, and know that you are more than just these feelings.

If you ask for help, it is given.

You cannot fail.

You are not alone.

WHAT DO WE NEED?

Once you've decided this person you love will live and die at home, choose the room or rooms that are most comfortable and convenient. Consider how much the person can move about and the location of bathrooms. Is the bedroom he or she used before still the favorite? Could you hear someone call from that room? Or would a bell or buzzer system be helpful? If a room was shared, do the people want to continue sharing it? Does the dying person like to be alone, or is a bed or couch in the living room, in the middle of the life-flow of the home, a desirable choice? Is there another place the family can be if the dying person wants to sleep or be alone? A cheerful, well-lit bedroom not far from the main living space and kitchen is a possibility—or even a greenhouse or porch depending on the weather.

It's helpful to position the bed to create easy access on both sides. This makes moving and turning the person and changing sheets easier. Bedside tables are useful for bottles, tissues, medical supplies, flowers, and other things you want handy.

Make a list of things you'll need and want, and go about getting them. Look around for what you can find at home. A list might go like this (not all are necessary, not even the first):

- A doctor (see the following section on finding a doctor)
- Prescribed medicines, particularly those for pain control
- A nurse
- A sense of humor
- A hospital bed, but only if both patient and family decide it would be easier. It's not always necessary and can be upsetting to the patient to give up his or her own bed even if a hospital bed might be more comfortable.
- A commode (potty chair), bedpan, or urinal. Commodes have a plastic can underneath that can be emptied. You can bring a bedpan or urinal home from the hospital or buy one. Urinals are for men only.
- A wheelchair, walker, crutches—according to the patient's needs
- Extra sheets and bedding. If you have a choice, choose designs and colors the person might like. Buy waterproof pads for beds and chairs. (Electric blankets are not recommended.)
- Extra nightgowns or pajamas that are easy to put on and take off. A nightshirt for man might be easier than pajamas. If you sew, you could copy a hospital gown in pleasing fabrics and colors.
- Bed jacket or cardigan sweater
- A glorious potted plant or bunches of wildflowers
- Massage lotion (try a health food store for natural products)
- A TV, VCR/DVD player, CD player, and/or radio

- Drinking straws that bend
- A cell phone or an extension on your telephone cord. It's ideal to have two telephones, one near the person (on which you can turn off the sound), and one to use in a place where you can talk privately.
- Extra pillows
- Alcohol, cotton balls, and hydrogen peroxide or swabs for teeth care
- A plastic dishpan for bathing
- Paper towels and tissues, and cotton towels
- Socks and nonskid slippers. Feet tend to get cold if the weather is at all cool.
- A stand-up bed tray if the person can feed him- or herself
- Two hot water bottles—one for the feet and one for easing pain

FINDING A DOCTOR

You need a doctor to assist the patient and family in making medical decisions, to prescribe medicines if necessary, and to authorize nursing services, insurance benefits, and hospice care. If the patient has to go into a hospital unexpectedly, a doctor can give directions that the patient's wishes in terms of treatment be respected. A doctor is useful for patient and family morale, although for day-to-day care a nurse may be more helpful.

You'll need a doctor who can understand the patient's desire to die at home and who is willing to support you. Try to find one who accepts death as a natural part of life. If you're able, discuss with the doctor how he or she feels about death and artificial means of prolonging life; then discuss how the dying person feels about these issues. This could save finding out later that the doctor you chose feels death is a personal or professional failure and will prolong a life no matter how inhumane the means or situation. When things are critical, there's no time for philosophical discussions.

A doctor who's willing to work with you as an equal and be personally involved in this dying process will be the most useful. She or he needs to be available for home visits and phone consultations. Doctoring partially by telephone can save a lot of wear and tear on everyone.

You may already have a doctor who fills the bill. If you have to find one, a hospice may be your best bet. Friends may recommend a doctor, or you may call a free clinic or university medical school. A growing number of young doctors are interested in home births and deaths. Call the local or county medical association and ask for a doctor who makes house calls. Look in the yellow pages under "physicians—general, family practice, or palliative care." Initial inquiries may be made by phone.

MOVING FROM HOSPITAL TO HOME

When the patient is ready and things are sorted out at home, you're ready for the next part of the adventure. If you're nervous, it's okay.

At any time, the patient, or the family at the patient's request, can check him- or herself out of the hospital. As mentioned earlier, it's easier if the doctor agrees, though it is very uncommon for one to try to stop someone from going home by instituting legal proceedings.

If the patient is taking medication or pain relievers, make arrangements with your doctor and have them available before you bring the patient home. If you will be responsible for giving injections immediately upon the patient's homecoming, get instructions, syringes, and needles beforehand.

Driving a person home in your car saves the cost of an ambulance. Use a wheelchair if necessary to move the patient to and from the car. If an ambulance is needed, again, be prepared to pay cash. The doctor may ask a nurse to call an ambulance, or you can call.

THE HOMECOMING

This may well be one of the most satisfying moments of the whole experience for you and the dying person. Homecoming with John, Mary, Dad, and Mom were times of joy and quiet satisfaction. Don't be discouraged if there are snags or difficulties. Both or all of you are learning and adjusting.

If there are children in the family, they may want to make their own kind of homecoming celebration. This is wonderful, as long as it's not too tiring for the home-comer. Joshua, Ben, and I made signs to welcome Dad when he came home from his chemotherapy weeks. Once, we dressed as clowns.

You've already completed some of the hardest work: making the decision and getting organized at home. You and the dying person are doing what feels right and are taking responsibility for your lives. The house probably feels peaceful and purposeful. The home-comer is often content or joyful and relieved to be in familiar surroundings. Even if it isn't their own home, it feels like a place for living. The dying person regains more ability to direct his or her own life.

My own experience with homecomings has been one of rightness (not righteousness) in cooperating with life by taking responsibility for dying. My feeling of helplessness vanished and was replaced by a sense of purposefulness. I was doing what I wanted to do, was being there for the person I loved, and it felt good. Feelings like this can carry you a long way through whatever lies ahead.

Sit down and put your feet up. Enjoy the satisfaction of your accomplishment and the beauty of home.

A human being is part of the whole, called by us the "Universe," a part limited in time and space. He experiences himself, his thoughts and feelings, as something separated from the rest—a kind of optical delusion of his consciousness. This delusion is a kind of prison for us, restricting us to our personal desires and to affection for a few persons nearest us. Our task must be to free ourselves from this prison by widening our circles of compassion to embrace all living creatures and the whole of nature in its beauty.

—Albert Einstein

6

MEDICAL CONSIDERATIONS

Too often we underestimate the power of a touch, a smile, a kind word, a listening ear, or the smallest act of caring, all of which have the potential to turn a life around.

—Leo F. Buscaglia

WHEN TO CALL A DOCTOR OR NURSE

You may find it surprising how little you need a doctor or nurse if you accept that the person you're caring for is dying. Much of what we need from the medical profession is moral support.

A doctor is properly called for counsel and assistance with some specific procedure, not to make decisions for you. Ask for help and guidance to make the dying process as comfortable as possible. Trust yourself and the dying person to make the choices and decisions that are best for you.

Call a doctor or nurse if you feel you're in over your head. Call if you feel you don't have sufficient knowledge to take responsibility for a decision. Call if you don't know what to do and panic, and the panic doesn't subside.

Other reasons for calling:

- complaints about pain
- breathing difficulties
- seizure
- developing bedsores
- catheter problems
- constipation
- bleeding

- drowsiness, confusion, or combativeness
- lack of urination
- unusual depression
- need for medication, supplies, or equipment
- the patient wants you to call

If you can't reach a doctor, call a nurse. In terms of practical care, a nurse is often more helpful than a doctor. If you're in a hospice program, call the nurse, who can call the doctor and get orders for pain medication or whatever else must be handled by a physician. Again, hospices direct families not to call 911 because doing so can result in the cancellation of your hospice benefit, and you may have to pay for alternative treatment.

There needs to be an explicit agreement about what the dying person wants the doctor to do. For example, a complication arises such as difficulty in breathing, perhaps due to pneumonia. Does the person want to be rushed to the hospital, which may prolong the dying process? In times past, pneumonia was called "The Old Man's Friend" because it can help a person to die. Is there a reason to cure it so the person can die later of cancer? There may be and there may not be. The point is that you discuss these scenarios with the dying person.

The dying person can share his or her wishes verbally with the doctor and ask that they be noted in his or her medical record. Hopefully, an advance directive such as a living will or durable power of attorney for health care has been signed (see chapter 11). If so, give the doctor a copy if you haven't already. The directive can be changed whenever the dying person chooses. Doctors feel freer to follow a patient's wishes if they know that the family understands that in a dying process, the dying person may die at any time and there is no blame.

Another way of ensuring that the dying person's wishes are carried out is to request a DNR, an acronym for "do not resuscitate," which affirms that the patient is not to be resuscitated in case of cardiac or respiratory arrest. This form can be signed at home or in the hospital by the patient, doctor, and a witness.

WORKING WITH A DOCTOR

If you are enrolled in a hospice program, you can count on the hospice doctor to be an invaluable ally in supporting your loved one in living fully until he or she dies. Many other doctors have also made peace with dying and will support you at home.

Taking time now to examine your relationship with doctors may help during this experience with dying and improve your relationships with them for the rest of your life.

Working with a doctor can teach us a lot about trusting and taking responsibility for ourselves and about how we relate to authority figures. Doctors are just ordinary people with a medical specialty. They have a difficult role in our society, as indicated by their unusually high incidence of suicide, drug addiction, and marital breakups.[1]

Often, we have set them up as gods, as knowers of mysteries we cannot hope to comprehend, and we feel cheated and angry if they can't heal us. It seems a little silly to make gods of specialists in livers or nostrils, and sillier still to turn our lives over to them. After years of working with people who expect them to be gods, many doctors start to believe it themselves. Then, when a patient dies, some take it as a personal failure—and we also see it as their personal failure.

Until recently, most of us have wanted doctors to be in control of our health. So they became habituated to being in charge and are sometimes astounded when someone wants to participate in his or her own health. A patient and family who want to are still often labeled "difficult." I suggest that it is better to be called "difficult" than to abdicate our responsibility, which may later cause us needless suffering.

Patients and families have generally reacted to doctors the same way people do to other authority figures—with feelings of hostility and/or intimidation. Neither attitude makes for an open, helpful relationship. In the long run it's not useful to have unrealistic expectations of doctors. Those expectations cause us disappointment and prevent doctors from being all of who they can be. It's not useful or accurate to assume, "The doctor knows and I don't." The most beneficial relationship between doctor, patient, and family might be a partnership of equals:

- The family and patient see doctors as helpers, feel compassion for them, and appreciate their expertise in an area (usually a limited one in terms of the total health picture).
- Doctors share their compassion and expertise with the family without suggesting they know all and the family knows nothing.
- The patient and family take responsibility for themselves and don't expect doctors to make life decisions about any life except their own.

A doctor's life would be a lot easier if he or she didn't feel responsible for the life of each patient; a doctor needs to be responsive to, not responsible for, a patient. When we feel responsible and things don't go as we'd like, we tend to feel guilty. Once we, as patients and families, get over the fright of not having someone else in charge, we'll feel a greater sense of responsibility for our own lives and increased confidence, power, and dignity. On the other hand, a doctor might find his or her life to be more meaningful if he or she is willing to be personally involved with patients and their families.

If, during this dying process, you have a problem getting your doctor to answer your questions and hear your concerns, be very direct. Often busy, harassed, and tired, doctors can seem like escape artists. You could say, "It seems like you're too busy to talk now. I'd like to make an appointment to talk about John's treatment."

Here are three questions to keep in mind when you talk with a doctor:

1. Presently, in simple terms, what's going on?
2. What do you think is best to do from here?
3. How much of this treatment is to keep this person alive, and how much is helping him or her to be comfortable?

After each question, repeat back to the doctor what was said to make sure you understand and to make sure everyone else knows you understand. Review the conversation. For example, "Did I understand correctly that you feel such and such?" You have a right to know what each treatment is for. And there is no shame in asking questions until you understand. Making notes can be helpful.

Write down medicines prescribed, then call a pharmacist and/or read about them in a standard drug book called the *Physician's Desk Reference* (PDR). The PDR is easily obtainable by non-physicians—your doctor may even give you last year's. You might also check your local library for *The Essential Guide to Prescription Drugs,* by James Rybacki.

The AMA 1986 policy statement that permits doctors to withhold all life-prolonging treatment from dying patients and the right-to-die laws have helped to alleviate the problem of doctors, with good intentions, resisting or obstructing a patient's right to die.

Those policies notwithstanding, you may sense that your doctor feels death is a personal failure, professional defeat, or a moral and legal dilemma instead of a natural event. If he or she is resisting or obstructing your loved one's right to die, you might discuss your feeling with him or her. Then, if death continues to be resisted, it may be time to get another doctor-helper.

Be aware that it's okay to change doctors or nurse-helpers if the dying person doesn't like the ones you have. Having people around us about whom we feel good is our right. This doesn't mean you need to pamper a *prima donna* patient who wants a new staff each day!

PHYSICAL PAIN AND PAIN RELIEVERS

The most consistently voiced fear about dying and death is physical pain, particularly in the case of cancer. You may be relieved to know that cancer is not necessarily painful. Some doctors estimate that 25 to 50 percent of advanced cancer patients experience no pain as a result of the cancer.[2] For patients who are in pain, its management is important to enable them to live fully until they die.

Each of us reacts differently to pain because it's experienced by the whole individual: physically, emotionally, mentally, and spiritually. A unique pain-relief program must be developed for each individual. With skilled help, we can control pain just as effectively at home as in a hospital. Nearly 90 percent of the time pain can be relieved with the right combination of medicine and dosing schedules.[3]

Even as we move to relieve pain, we need to be aware of its purpose. Pain is neither good nor bad; it's simply a messenger that tells us something in our lives or bodies is not working and needs attention. It's generally pain that moves us to leave behind old patterns and ways of being that no longer work. The more a dying person clings to the body, the more pain she or he experiences.

Perhaps the role that physical pain plays in the dying process is to loosen our attachment to our bodies and dispel the illusion that we are our bodies: “Hey, my body is getting uninhabitable. I need to consider getting out of here.” Be aware that there is an “I” apart from the body. Without a body, there is no pain. Death itself is painless. Getting ready for it, however, can be painful.

Dying people may be afraid to admit they're in pain, feeling ashamed of being “weak,” or afraid of addiction or returning to the hospital. Encourage them to speak up and not to “tough it out,” so they can use their energy to live well until they die. Having pain does not indicate weakness, just *humanness.* Suffering is not noble. Let the person know pain can be controlled at home so they needn't fear returning to a hospital. Reassure them that the therapeutic aim in their case is pain relief and addiction is not a concern.

Sudden, unexpected pain, called *acute pain,* causes anxiety. Your attitude toward pain can do much to help the person experiencing it. Your fear and resistance to their pain increases their fear and resistance, and their fear and resistance increases their pain. You can help by not saying, for example, “Oh, pain, terrible. We've got to get rid of it right away!” Allow the person to learn what he or she can from it as you quietly move toward relieving it, if that's the person's choice. Do what the dying person wants. No human being should be degraded by having to beg for pain relief.

You might try using the word *sensation* instead of *pain.* Taking the label off pain often changes our experience of it. Aspirin and different strengths of Tylenol can be used for non-severe acute pain. If there is severe pain for which you are unprepared, call your doctor or nurse.

Pain that endures over time is called *chronic.* Chronic pain experienced by a dying person can generally be relieved. Because we want to live until we die, it's important to know that alertness and chronic pain relief can be balanced. To be conscious at death is a choice similar to being conscious for birth pains. Some women like to be unconscious and wake up with a baby beside them; others prefer to be awake, cooperating with and participating in the experience. Perhaps dying is the labor pain of the soul. Some may not care if they're unconscious, and others prefer to be present for their dying. It's a personal choice. There's no right or wrong way. Either way works.

Whatever the pain challenge, the patient and doctor decide together which drug or combination of drugs might be most suitable. A pain reliever that works for one person may not work for another. A dosage therapeutic for one may be toxic for another. Consider drug allergies. (John Muir, for example, was allergic to opium and its derivatives, which include many commonly used narcotics.) A person may have to try a number of alternatives until pain relief and alertness are balanced. In the words of Ivan Illich, we don't want to turn "patients into pets," as many nursing homes do.[4]

The secret of chronic pain relief is regularity. Pain relievers should be given at regular intervals before the pain begins, and the dosage should be adjusted to handle the entire period. Machos and stoics do themselves and their families a disservice by waiting until they're in agony to take pain medication. Pain is much more difficult to control if it's very severe before medication is given.

A person skilled in pain management needs to set up the time schedule, which can of course be changed at any time to meet the patient's needs. Ask the patient to keep you advised of how she or he feels.

There are a number of ways pain medications can be administered: orally (pill or liquid), intravenously (injections), subcutaneously (pumps), transdermally (skin patches), and with suppositories. There are many pain relievers, from analgesics such as aspirin and Tylenol to narcotics or opioids such as codeine, morphine, oxycodone (Percodan, Percocet,

Tylox), methadone, Dilaudid, and fentanyl. The appropriate one to use is the one that alleviates the pain, which is determined by the severity of the pain and the patient's tolerance.

Many hospices use liquid morphine to effectively control pain for dying patients, particularly "breakthrough pain," sudden intense pain that is not alleviated by a patient's regular pain medication. Its chief advantages are that it's easy to take and enters the bloodstream quickly. The morphine solution is usually given every four hours around the clock. There are also long-acting morphine tablets, which last twelve hours, that may be given before bedtime to eliminate waking the dying person and yourself in the middle of the night.

The side effects of oral morphine and most narcotic pain relievers are nausea, constipation, and sleepiness. Nausea can be treated with anti-nausea agents such as Compazine, taken about a half hour before the pain reliever. Constipation can be remedied a number of ways. (In this chapter, see the section on constipation.)

Narcotic means "sleep inducing." During the first few days of taking a narcotic, a person may feel drowsy. As the body adjusts and the person catches up on sleep lost while in pain, she or he usually becomes alert again and may live fully the remaining time. If drowsiness continues, the dosage can be adjusted. Narcotics can be combined with Tylenol, aspirin, non-steroidal anti-inflammatories (for example, Motrin), or antidepressants to maximize pain control and minimize sleepiness. Sometimes prednisone is given once a day in the morning to enhance the patient's appetite and sense of well-being.

If the dying person can no longer swallow or is vomiting, injections, transdermal patches, or suppositories may be substituted. While transdermal patches are easy to apply, their downside is that dosage levels can't be controlled. And here's a tip from a hospice nursing director: you can coat any pain pill with Vaseline and insert it like a suppository.

A fairly common form of pain control is the use of pumps to administer the desired drug. Often called PCAs, or patient-controlled analgesia devices, these pumps are worn at the waist and deliver a constant flow of morphine, for example, through a plastic tube to a small hypodermic needle usually implanted under the skin of the chest. Family or the patient can push a button to increase the dosage of pain medication.

The pump is useful for people for whom other forms of pain control haven't worked, and especially for people whose stomachs or intestines have been severely damaged. You might want to ask a hospice doctor, medical oncologist, or a pain clinic connected to a hospital or doctor's group if this option is available.

A new development for breakthrough pain is Actiq, a sweetened lozenge on a stick, packed with fentanyl, which can be rubbed on the inside of the cheek to rush opioids to the brain. Patients report getting relief using Actiq in as little as five minutes.

Whatever pain reliever, or relievers, you use for your loved ones, *pay attention* and stay flexible. For example, a doctor may say one shot should last five hours. The patient reports that it lasts only three. Consult with your hospice nurse or doctor about changing the dosage.

Hospices will often give families an emergency kit of medicines to control severe pain until a nurse can get to you. This saves you unnecessary stress if severe pain occurs in the middle of the night. If you're not enrolled in a hospice program, you may want to ask your doctor to give you a prescription for a medication for unexpected severe pain and purchase it ahead of time.

In appendix A, you will find a hospice standing order form similar to those used by many hospices. Standing orders are doctors' instructions used by hospice nurses for routine medical concerns. You may want to check it to learn about specific things you can use, or do, to help your patient.

Listed below are commonly used medical abbreviations, which will help you to understand the often mysterious letters that appear on doctors' orders and prescriptions.

Commonly Used Medical Abbreviations

Abbreviation	Meaning
• a	• Before
• a.c.	• Before food or meals
• ad lib.	• To the amount desired
• b.i.d., b.d.	• Two times a day
• b.i.n., b.n.	• Two times a night
• b.m.r.	• Basal metabolic rate
• b.p.	• Blood pressure
• c.	• With
• e.g.	• For example
• ext.	• Extract
• fl.	• Fluid
• gtt (s).	• A drop, drops
• h., hr.	• Hour
• h.s.	• At bedtime
• I.M.	• Intramuscular
• I.V.	• Intravenous
• noct.	• At night
• NPO	• Nothing by mouth
• p.o.	• Give orally
• p.r.n.	• As needed
• q.d.	• Every day

• q.i.d.	• Four times a day
• q.o.d.	• Every other day
• Sx	• Symptoms
• t.i.d.	• Three times a day
• Tx	• Treatments
• U.S.P. U.S.	• Pharmacopoeia

ALTERNATIVES TO MEDICALLY APPROVED PAIN MEDICATIONS

There are a number of alternatives to medically used drugs: whiskey or other strong spirits, biofeedback, heat, massage, acupuncture, hypnosis, color therapy, LSD, marijuana, mescaline, and laughing gas—or laughing. The appropriate choice is determined by the dying person and influenced by the content and style of life before the illness.

Marijuana, mescaline, and LSD have been used experimentally with the dying process. The fear and hysteria built up around these drugs have obscured their useful medical qualities. The active ingredient of marijuana, THC, has proved effective in preventing nausea in chemotherapy patients. It acts as a mood elevator and tranquilizer, tends to retard weight loss by stimulating the appetite, and potentiates pain medications so that less is needed.

Mescaline and LSD, consciousness-expanding drugs, seem to enlarge the framework in which a person experiences pain, changing the experience of it and sometimes eliminating pain entirely. Laura Huxley in *This Timeless Moment* describes the death of Aldous Huxley, an innovative adventurer in the human mind. Huxley used LSD in his last days in order to experience his death as fully as possible.

Stanislav Grof and a group at the Maryland Psychiatric Research Center, doing research on cancer and LSD, made an interesting pain discovery. Grof and Joan Halifax reported in their book *Human Encounter with Death* that pain is relieved by a "transpersonal experience": a mystical experience in which one goes beyond the usual limits of personality and connects with some large whole, perhaps God.[5] (See chapter 12 for one technique for guiding someone into a transcendent space without drugs.)

Charles Grob, MD, a UCLA psychiatrist, has recently been experimenting with psilocybin, a mushroom derivative, to reduce anxiety, which could be a useful therapeutic tool for people experiencing severe anxiety in the dying process.

Breathing and visualization techniques can be very useful non-chemical ways of working with pain. If there's delay in getting a pain reliever, you might try them. In some cases, they may preclude the need for drugs at all. Breathing can be as useful for dying as it is for birthing. When we feel pain, we tense up and tend to stop breathing fully. Our cells don't get the oxygen they need to clean out toxins and keep the nerve signals straight, and the pain gets worse.

One of the first things to do for pain is to *keep breathing.* Unless someone has had previous experience with breathing consciously, he or she may focus on the pain and fear and forget to breathe. As the helper, encourage the person to breathe deeply, to breathe into the area that hurts, and then to breathe down into the toes. Ask the person to relax, to "soften" around the area that hurts, and open him- or herself to the sensation of pain. As the person surrenders, gives up resistance, more oxygen enters the area and the pain may lessen. The body senses that its message is received and relaxes. Keep repeating "soften, relax, open."

Paying attention to pain helps relieve it as long as we don't judge it as bad! Pain just exists; it is not inherently good or bad.

I have found it helpful to combine breathing techniques with hot water bottles and foot massages. While the person is breathing into the area that hurts, partially fill two hot water bottles with hot, not boiling, water. Cover the bottles with a towel so you don't burn the person's skin, and place them under the feet and on the area that hurts. If you don't have hot water bottles, put the person's feet into a bucket of medium-hot tap water. Put a hot washcloth on the forehead. Together these seem to keep energy moving through the body so pain is lessened or eliminated. Some people prefer ice packs and cold water; either is okay. If it feels right to you, add a foot massage to further relax the person and to stimulate increased circulation. Breathing and foot massage are useful techniques for calming *anyone* in a stressful situation. You might want to take time for them yourself.

I have heard talk in natural healing circles that taking drugs for pain is somehow not spiritual. That's baloney. Again, physical pain is a message that something's not working right in the body. The dying get the message loud and clear, only this time there's nothing they can do about it. The body can't be fixed. Taking drugs frees us to experience dying on levels other than the body. If dying teaches us anything, it teaches us that we're more than just a body. However, if we're in pain, the body commands our undivided attention.

If, as many people believe, our essential identity is God, why torture God's body—or anyone else's—by not taking pain medication? That's cruelty. If we truly believe that everything is equally sacred, morphine is just as sacred as the herb from which it's derived.

SHOTS OR INJECTIONS

There are two types (routes) of shots or injections used for giving pain relievers: intravenous, in which the solution is injected directly into a vein, and intramuscular, in which it's injected into muscle tissue. Intravenous shots should be given only by a qualified doctor, nurse, or medic. If necessary, you can give intramuscular ones. Ask a doctor or nurse to show you how and practice ahead of time on an orange. The following instructions and diagram will help you as well.

Don't panic. Giving an intramuscular shot is not difficult or dangerous, although it may be frightening to think about. You will likely forget your fear if someone you love is suffering in front of you and you know you can do something about it. Remember, love transforms fear.

Have the prescribed drug(s) and the correct-size syringes and needles available. If you've had experience in giving shots, you can protect a person's privacy by giving it in the arm or upper thigh. If you haven't, it's best to use the buttock.

Preparing and Giving an Intramuscular Injection

1. Position the person comfortably to receive the injection and ask him or her to relax. If administering to the buttock, ask the person to turn the toes inward to relax the muscle. (The discomfort of intramuscular shots is usually due to tension in muscle tissue.)
2. Swab the bottle top with alcohol. If you use an ampoule, hold the top with a paper towel and break if off, holding the base firmly and snapping the top toward you.

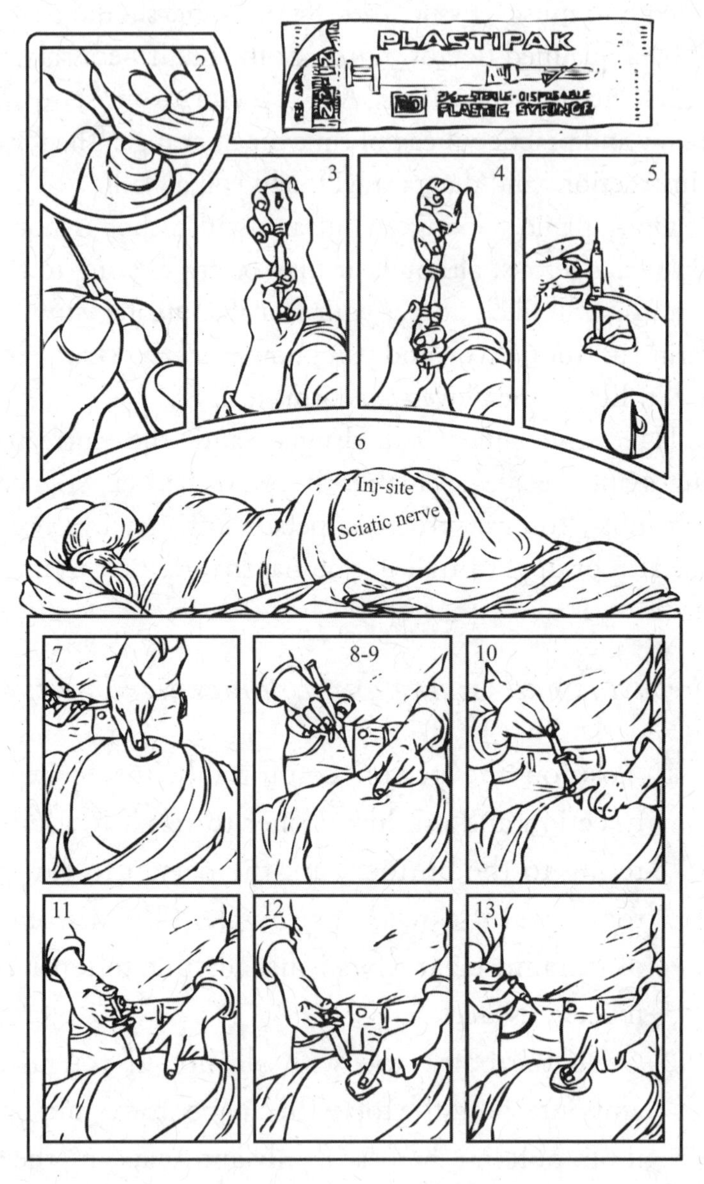

How to Give an Intramuscular Injection

Remove the sterile syringe and needle from the package and check that the needle is secure. If the syringe and needle are separate, screw them together without touching the metal needle.

3. Insert the needle into the bottle or ampoule. (For a bottle only, first inject air into it—the same amount as the dose of medication. If you want 1 cc. out of the bottle, inject 1 cc. of air into it first.)

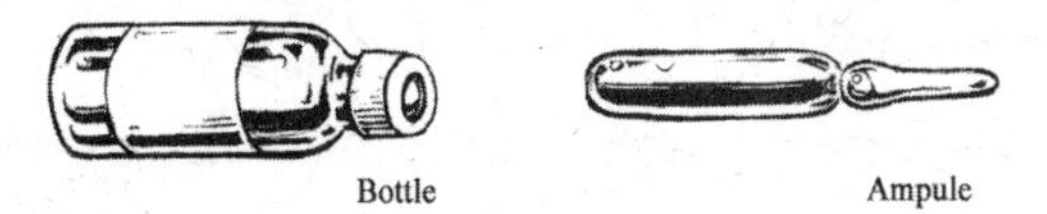

4. Pull the plunger until the correct dosage is shown on the syringe scale and remove the needle from the bottle or ampoule.
5. With needle end pointed up, tap the syringe with your finger and push in the plunger slightly to remove excess air. (Don't worry about injecting small air bubbles with an intramuscular injection. It may be uncomfortable, but isn't dangerous.) It's okay if a little of the solution spurts out of the needle.
6. Choose an injection site in the upper outer quadrant of either buttock (see diagram). This is important to avoid the sciatic nerve or a large blood vessel.
7. Thoroughly clean the injection site using a prepared swab or a cotton ball saturated with alcohol.
8. With the thumb and first finger of your free hand, press down, spreading the skin around the site.
9. Hold the syringe up and, like a dart, quickly and deliberately thrust the needle into the buttock at a ninety-degree angle. (You'll find this doesn't rule out gentleness.)
10. With the needle in place, pull back the plunger slightly to see if any blood appears in the syringe.

If it does, you've hit a vein and must remove the needles and choose a new site.

11. Inject the medicine slowly.
12. Quickly remove the needle, and then apply gentle pressure on the site with the cotton ball or prepared alcohol swab.
13. Massage the area gently and firmly to help the medicine be absorbed.
14. Destroy the used needle by bending and breaking it. Do not touch the needle after using it, especially if you are injecting someone who has a communicable disease. Some pharmacies sell inexpensive needle disposers, which are useful if you give injections often.

IVS AND DEHYDRATION

The question of intravenous feeding (through IVs) may come up for you. IVs are used to nourish people who can't eat or drink enough to stay alive. The decision whether or not to use IVs in terminal care raises again the issue of the quality of life versus the quantity. Feeding the body cells by means of IVs often prolongs the life of the body. The cost is discomfort, less ability to move, and the need to have a nurse. Dad said, "When I've got those tubes in I feel like a patient. When I don't, I feel like me."

The result of not taking enough fluids into the body is dehydration. The chemical imbalance created by lack of fluids often causes a person to have a sense of well-being or euphoria. As I said earlier, reportedly it's a relatively comfortable death. The main discomfort—dryness of the mouth and thirst—is helped by sucking on ice chips and clean, moistened washcloths. It generally takes only a few days for a debilitated person to die from lack of fluids.

If someone has not yet accepted that she or he is dying and wants to be fed intravenously, a doctor or nurse can show you how IVs work and what problems to watch for. There can be local pain and inflammation at the needle site. The needle can slip out of the vein, causing the liquid to fill the surrounding tissue. A qualified nurse needs to start the IV and to come by often to check it. Bottles are changed three to six times a day.

Don't worry if a bottle runs out. Air is not going to get in and kill the person. If the fluid is not running, a clot forms around the needle, and the needle then has to be changed. Ask the nurse ahead of time what to do if the tubing falls out, comes apart, or has air bubbles.

One of the most common fears people have about shots and IVs is that air will get in and kill the person. Actually, a surprisingly large amount of air has to go directly into a vein or artery before there's a problem.

SKIN CARE AND BEDSORES

Skin care is important medically as well as to help a person maintain dignity and comfort. If the skin is not properly cared for, bedsores can result. Bedsores (decubitus ulcers) are caused when skin tissue breaks down.

The first sign of skin breakdown is red, sore areas. They occur where prolonged pressure limits circulation of oxygen to the skin. Uncared for, they can become painful, oozing, raw areas where infection can set in. The best thing to do about bedsores is to prevent them from occurring in the first place. The less a person can move, the greater the chance they will develop bedsores.

The areas to watch for possibly developing bedsores are elbows, inner knees, back of the head and ears, shoulders, lower back and buttocks, and heels.

You can prevent bedsores by turning a person in bed at least every couple of hours, massaging the skin to keep blood circulating in the area, drying the skin well after bathing, and exposing the skin to air. Before bedsores appear, use a Therm-a-Rest mattress topper, a sheepskin pad, or an egg-crate mattress (a foam pad with indentations like an egg box) under the person. Hospices often use adjustable, electric alternating pressure pads that fit over the bed and which you can buy from a medical supply company. You may not need one to prevent bedsores if the person is massaged and turned frequently, but they are comfortable.

To protect the coccyx (tailbone), you can place a four-inch foam cushion on a wheelchair or other hard seat. It's helpful to place a soft cloth or pillow between the knees of someone who is lying on his or her side and is confined to bed. Body surfaces that touch can cause pressure, friction, and skin breakdown. You may also buy toughening creams that contain a tincture of benzoic acid to protect the skin (Lanacaine, Solarcaine, etc.) or a medicated cream ordered by a doctor.

The basic idea is this: if the skin is wet, dry it; if it's too dry, moisten it. Use a light skin oil to keep the skin supple. To keep the skin dry, use a drying cream such as Desitin, or powders such as Johnson's Baby Powder or Mexana. Obviously, any area exposed to urine needs to be washed and dried well.

To prevent bedsores, many hospices use Stomahesive wafers and/or DuoDERM dressings. These Band-Aid-like dressings act like a second skin to prevent breakdown. Place a Stomahesive wafer, for example, on skin that remains reddened over the coccyx, ankles, knees, or hips. If the skin has already broken down—if it looks mottled, black, or like an abrasion—use a DuoDERM dressing. Both are available at medical supply companies or at some drug stores.

If areas of the skin do redden and break down, be sure to show the doctor or nurse and ask for suggestions.

ELIMINATION AND INCONTINENCE

Often a person who is very ill or very old will have problems with elimination. As diet changes and a person exercises less, organs are weakened and the bowels and bladder start loosening or become blocked. "Incontinence" means loss of bladder or bowel control. Losing control over elimination, one of the most basic life functions, can be very demoralizing. A person experiencing this loss needs our compassion and caring to adjust. (See the section on elimination in chapter 9 for ways to assist the person physically and emotionally.)

Catheters

A catheter is a flexible tube inserted into the urethra (the canal that takes urine out of the body) and is usually connected to a plastic sack at the other end. It's used when bladder control is lost and can help prevent skin deterioration due to wetness. For men, there is a catheter that fits on the outside of the penis like a sheath called a condom catheter. You'll need instructions from a nurse in the use and care of catheters and things to watch for, such as infection.

An alternative for dealing with lost bladder control is disposable cotton pads or diapers (again, see the chapter 9 section on elimination).

Tell the dying person about the alternatives and ask for their preference. Some people find catheters uncomfortable.

Constipation

A blockage in the bowels can cause discomfort and pain and eventually may be life-threatening. Paying attention to and treating constipation is an important part of home care, particularly if your patient is taking pain-relief drugs that cause constipation. A general rule of thumb is to use a laxative or enema if there has been no bowel movement for three days.

If the patient has undiagnosed abdominal pain, check with your doctor.

Natural ways to deal with constipation are activity, a diet adequate in fiber, drinking lots of water, coffee or some herbal teas, and using a toilet or potty chair instead of a bedpan. A diet containing bran, lots of fresh vegetables, and fruits and their juices (prune and apple particularly) is helpful. White bread, white rice, meat, and cheese tend to cause constipation.

Acidophilus and probiotics—natural intestinal flora—help relieve constipation and diarrhea by reestablishing the balance of intestinal bacteria, which is very important for people whose own intestinal bacteria have been killed by antibiotics or chemotherapy. Yogurt contains acidophilus. Probiotics are available at health food stores in tablets or liquid form.

Temporary constipation may be relieved by a natural laxative such as Nature's Way or a bulk-forming laxative like Metamucil. For chronic constipation, try a combination of stool softener and bowel stimulant such as Colace or Senokot-S (no prescription required). If more stimulation is needed, you can add Dulcolax tablets or suppositories to the above. Some hospices use Colace, a stool softener, and lactulose or two tablespoons of milk of magnesia before bedtime.

An enema is a simple procedure many of us have already used for constipation. You can buy a disposable premixed one, such as Fleets Enema, or mix one yourself. Here's a recipe: Dissolve two or three tablespoons of honey or one tablespoon of castile soap with enough water to fill an enema bag, or fill the bag with coffee or comfrey tea (drinking strength). Place a disposable pad under the person. Put Vaseline or cream around the tip to be inserted into the rectum.

Roll the person onto his or her left side and gently insert the tip three or four inches into the rectum. Hold the bag eighteen to twenty-four inches above the person's hip and allow the water to flow slowly into the colon. Lowering the bag slows down the flow. Ask the person to breathe deeply and relax and to hold the solution as long as possible. When the person can't hold it any longer and needs to let go, use a bedpan if getting to the bathroom or potty chair isn't possible. Be sure to wash and powder the area afterward, and then wash your own hands.

If the person fails to respond to a laxative or enema, a nurse or doctor will have to do a digital de-impaction, which means digging the stool out by hand with gloves on. An impaction is painful and unpleasant. It usually won't occur if you pay attention to constipation; however, I had to do one for Mom several times.

Diarrhea

Diarrhea is the body's way of getting rid of something it doesn't want—in a hurry. Unless it continues and/or the patient is getting weak from dehydration, it's often best to let it run its course. Cooked food, including white rice, tends to slow down diarrhea, as do bananas and gelatin. Acidophilus and probiotics will help rebalance the intestinal tract bacteria.

If these don't work, simple diarrhea is easily treated with Kaopectate and Pepto-Bismol. If it proves more difficult to treat, you'll need a prescription for something like Lomotil, paregoric, or codeine.

Sometimes a little diarrhea is a sign that stool is blocking the intestine. Liquid passes around the stool, and it appears to be diarrhea. If a person's fluid intake and movement are limited, and/or they're taking narcotic drugs and the bowel has not moved normally, give an enema. Unless there is severe abdominal pain, it can't hurt and may clear the blockage.

If there is severe abdominal pain, call your hospice nurse or doctor.

INSOMNIA

The cares and concerns of a dying person may cause sleeplessness. If your patient has difficulty sleeping, see if you can help without sleeping pills and barbiturates. Addiction is not a real concern with the dying, but why interfere more with delicate body balances? Some possibilities are to take, before bedtime, calcium tablets (two grams), chamomile tea, valerian tablets, a warm glass of milk, or tryptophan. Tryptophan is an amino acid in meat, milk, and cheese. Turkey is high in tryptophan. (Remember how tired you felt after Thanksgiving dinner?) Try a warm bath, hot foot bath, a back rub, or foot massage.

Stroke the hair and scalp and encourage the person to let all thoughts float away and let the head feel spacious and empty, clouds drifting in and out. When I can't sleep, I use the Bach flower remedy "sweet chestnut" or Tylenol PM.

Avoid coffee, black tea, and all dark-colored colas before bedtime. They contain eye-opening caffeine.

It's also okay not to go to sleep even when someone else thinks it time. Encourage the person to read, write, watch TV, listen to soothing music, or think for a while. If not sleeping continues to trouble the patient, ask a doctor about sleeping medications. Hospices often use 25 mg of Benadryl.

FEVER

If the patient starts to run a fever, you can treat it with aspirin unless he or she is allergic. Tylenol is preferable if the stomach is upset or the patient has a problem with ulcers or bleeding. A tepid or lukewarm sponge bath can be very effective in reducing a child's fever. For a high fever, you can wrap a child or adult in cold wet sheets and cover them with blankets. If the fever continues or increases, you may want to call a doctor.

DEPRESSION

A dying person may experience depression. For the useful role it plays in the dying process, see the chapter 7 section on Dr. Kübler-Ross's stages of dying. Depression tends not to be as long lasting or severe at home because the person has more control over his or her life. If depression persists, the person may need help with counseling or mood-elevating drugs. I have yet to see severe depression during a home dying.

Depression causes actual chemical changes in the body. Chronic pain can wear us down until we feel depressed and hopeless. These feelings may lift when the pain is relieved; however, some people become habituated to depression and it persists. To break the cycle, try to help the person refocus their energy. Because depression is often a result of not expressing what we feel, encourage the person to express sadness or whatever they're feeling and to live fully the time they have.

Some people may want to temporarily combine a pain reliever with an antidepressant. Elavil, Sinequan, and Paxil are commonly prescribed antidepressants. Funny movies or stories may also help. I use Bach flower remedies.

Sometimes depression is a side effect of pain medications. Have your doctor change the pain medication or combine it with one of the antidepressants mentioned above.

DEMENTIA OR IRRATIONALITY

Dementia is the Latin word for "irrationality." It's a temporary or permanent loss of connection to the generally accepted reality. You may not encounter it. I have a number of times, as a result of overmedication. If you do, attempt to find the cause or unexpressed need behind it. If possible, change the condition or meet the need.

Irrationality may be a result of pain, overmedication, exhaustion, blockage in the colon, or emotional frustration.

In these cases, you can often reverse the cause. Sometimes it helps to change the person's physical position: for example, from lying in bed to sitting up in a wheelchair. Suggest a walk if it's possible.

Irrationality may not be reversible in the case of senility, Alzheimer's, or a brain tumor. Not all brain tumors cause irrationality. It depends on the part of the brain that is affected.

If a person experiencing irrationality who also can't walk tries to get out of bed, hold them gently and firmly, talk with them, massage them, or do whatever occurs to you to do that calmly redirects their attention. For their own protection, they may need to be physically restrained. You can use a restraining chair: a wheelchair with a tray that locks into place. If the person's in bed, fold a sheet until it's one-foot wide, place it across the chest and arms, and tuck it snugly under the mattress on both sides. Your doctor or nurse can also advise you about different types of restraints.

For severe agitation or hysteria, which I've not yet seen in people dying at home, tranquilizing medication may be necessary. Haldol, Thorazine, and Navane are sometimes used. I regard them as a last resort when we've exhausted every other possibility. I would use them *only* to protect someone from harming themselves or others. Again, we don't want to turn patients into pets.

If a person with dementia is sitting around not harming anyone and rambling to him- or herself, the only change necessary may be in our attitude. Irrationality may serve a useful purpose in the dying process by allowing a person to disconnect from this reality and to prepare for the next. If it's painful for you to witness, allow your sadness and remember that we don't all have to have the same reality, and we can and should respect another's. It can be interesting and helpful to enter the world of someone we've judged to be irrational and see what we can learn.

⁂

Situations other than those I've discussed may arise and can also be taken care of at home. For example, if the dying person needs oxygen for comfort, you can rent an "oxygen concentrator." It's a little machine that gathers oxygen from the air, concentrates it, and delivers it to the person through nose tubes or a face mask.

If the person is choking on secretions, your hospice will have a portable suction machine, or you can rent one from a medical supply store. There's even one kind of suction machine patients can use on themselves. A nurse can show you how to use these.

Some other possibilities are included in the hospice physician's standing orders sample form (see appendix A). If you are not in a hospice program, you might want to share it with your doctor.

If the person you're caring for has AIDS, they need the same loving care as anyone else. You will need to take extra precautions to prevent infection to yourself or to the person with AIDS. In a dying situation, prevention requires not coming into direct contact with blood. HIV/AIDS is not passed through saliva, tears, sweat, feces, or urine. The Center for Disease Control and Prevention (CDC) has an excellent web site that gives all the information you need to care for someone with AIDS, from how to wash the sheets and dispose of needles to respite care and socializing.

PRAYER FOR PEACE

(A version of the Prayer of St. Francis sent to me by Mother Teresa.)

Lord, make me a channel for your peace that
Where there is hatred, I may bring love
Where there is wrong, I may bring the
spirit of forgiveness
Where there is discord, I may bring harmony
Where there is error, I may bring truth
Where there is doubt, I may bring faith
Where there is despair, I may bring hope
Where there are shadows, I may bring light
Where there is sadness, I may bring joy
Lord, grant that I may seek rather to comfort
than to be comforted
To understand than to be understood
To love than to be loved
For it is by forgetting self that one finds
It is in forgiving that one is forgiven
It is by dying that one awakes to the eternal.
AMEN

God bless you
M Teresa MC

7

BEING WITH SOMEONE WHO IS DYING

The first duty of love is to listen.

—Paul Tillich

ELISABETH KÜBLER-ROSS' STAGES OF DYING

Elisabeth Kübler-Ross, a Swiss-born doctor and author of *On Death and Dying,* has served us all with great love. Her work with dying people and the attitude she brought to dying have given many people all over the world the courage to examine a part of our lives that we've not faced before. Working with hundreds of patients, she noted a process that most go through as they die. Most people don't consciously want to die, and this process is the way in which they make peace with this change.

The stages—denial and isolation, anger, bargaining, depression, and acceptance—are a process, not a goal. It's the same process many of us go through in facing any loss. Not all people go through all the stages; some skip stages and others move back and forth between them, sometimes from moment to moment.

The following description of the stages is just a clue to feelings you and the dying person may have. If our choice is to let people die in their own way, there's no need to push them through the stages to acceptance. A person can die with dignity even if he or she never accepts dying.

Denial and Isolation

Dr. Kübler-Ross called this the "No, not me" stage. It appears in the beginning of a life-threatening illness and often reappears many times. "It can't be true," is the patient's mantra, and he or she may shop around for different doctors or treatments. She or he may not want to "talk about it" or may want to be alone or with people who don't know what's happening. Shock and numbness are common. Dr. Kübler-Ross suggests that we just be there lovingly when a person is denying and let them know, "When you want to talk, I'm available."

A person may need denial to cope with impending death, to adjust to losses already experienced, and to tolerate suffering or pain. Some die in denial—that's their way. As family and friends, we may also experience denial. Check to see if the denial is yours or the dying person's.

Anger

The "Why Me?" stage, which is filled with rage, envy, and resentment. Anger is randomly projected, often on innocent people: "You don't love me." "The doctors and nurses are incompetent." "Goddamn, God!" Dr. Kübler-Ross suggests we not respond with nasty criticism, nor kill our loved one with kindness. It's better to rub it in. Affirm what's happening: "Doesn't it make you mad?" "Don't you feel like screaming?" The relief from venting anger may move the person toward greater acceptance of what is happening.

Sometimes the most loving thing we can do for a dying person is to be a target for an outburst of anger. It's not hard to do if we don't take it personally and remember that expressing anger often helps a person move toward accepting dying. I'm not suggesting, however, that you be a patsy for an angry bully.

It's okay to feel scared if the person yells at you, and it's okay to be angry with God. Imagining yourself in their place may help you understand their fears and anger. You might be angry too!

Bargaining

The "Yes, me, but..." stage. "It's okay for me to die if I can just make a trip to Hawaii first." "If I can just live till the kids graduate..." "If I live, I'll dedicate my life to God." Bargaining is a temporary truce. The patient may seem peaceful. It's a good time to take care of wills and other business. Dr. Kübler-Ross notes that very few people keep their bargains if they do live longer.

Depression

The "Yes, me" stage. Dr. Kübler-Ross talks about two kinds of depression: reactive, for loss of job, a breast, the ability to take care of oneself; and preparatory, preparing for the loss of life and family. The dying person needs time to be alone during this stage to make the emotional preparations. This can be a good time for quiet hand-holding.

Depression is the womb in which a new choice or way of being grows. It's caused by holding on to someone or something we can't have or by holding in some feeling we haven't expressed: anger, sadness, guilt, even love. One form of depression is "trapped love." We feel depressed when we block ourselves from receiving or expressing the living love that we are.

Depression is useful for a dying person and family holding on to a body. Making a change or letting go eventually becomes more desirable than the grayness of depression. You may be able to help someone see which feeling needs expressing.

Acceptance

The "It's okay; I'm ready for whatever comes" stage. The person is quiet, at peace, neither depressed nor angry. Dr. Kübler-Ross describes it as "time to contemplate the coming end with a certain degree of quiet expectation." The person is probably sleeping more; his or her concerns no longer relate to the outside world. It is "the final rest before a long journey." This period may be almost void of feeling. You can be there for him or her quietly, reassuringly.

Our response to dying is like any other big decision we make in our lives. We can go from acceptance, having made a decision, back into questioning that decision. It's very helpful to look for this process in ourselves as well as in the dying person we love. It's important for the family to arrive at acceptance so their desire to prolong life doesn't contradict the patient's wish to die in peace. It's easier if we feel acceptance when we bring someone home, even if this feeling changes many times.

TELLING SOMEONE THEY MAY DIE

In the past, many doctors, with good intentions, thought it kinder to alleviate a dying person's confusion by not speaking about dying. Now more doctors are straightforward in speaking with their terminally ill patients. If your doctor is not, however, you may want to talk with him or her about it.

If we avoid telling someone the facts, we're assuming responsibility for his or her life. We can be responsive to another person; we cannot be responsible for them. If a person wants to deny they're dying, that's their right. It's not our right, however, to take it upon ourselves to make that decision for them. If we don't tell someone, we are denying them the opportunity to get their affairs in order and to do things they've wanted to do, which might help them prepare for dying. We deny them the opportunity to try alternative treatments. It's more stressful to wonder if you're dying than to know.

I worried about telling someone they were dying when I began to be around people who were dying. Like most things we worry about, it didn't materialize in any way I had imagined.

The first time I told someone she was dying, it was indirectly and accidentally. A nurse at the hospital asked me to talk with a cancer patient who was dying and feeling depressed. I'll call her Rosa. I asked two nurses if Rosa knew she had cancer and was dying. Both said yes.

I talked with Rosa about her life and cancer. I left her feeling good about the visit. Communication had been opened, and I'd told her I'd be back to see her later. The next thing I heard about Rosa was that the head nurse and doctor were in a rage about "some idiot in the Pastoral Care and Counseling Department" (me, as it turned out), and Rosa was furious! The doctor hadn't told her she had cancer or was dying. He felt she was too sick and would take the news badly! I got through all the anger directed at me without feeling terrible by remembering that I'd done what seemed appropriate at the time, and also that expressing anger could help Rosa accept dying. Unfortunately, I was forbidden to see her again.

Generally, the doctor will tell a person that she or he is dying. The doctor is the appropriate person to deliver the news of a possibly fatal diagnosis because he or she is *believable* on the subject of physical death.

Optimally, the doctor will have spent some time with the person and will be aware of how she or he is handling illness. The doctor may then sensitively give the person information about the disease and its possible or probable outcome *as the doctor sees it.* You can discuss with the doctor how this might be done best. It's very important that the doctor not take away all sense of hope. (See the section on hope in chapter 10.)

The doctor might say, "At this point your medical situation looks difficult. I don't know anything we can do medically to cure you, but we can make you comfortable. It's always possible you'll have a remission or a new treatment will become available." Leave room for miracles. They happen.

Once a possibly fatal diagnosis is given, there's no need to try to force someone to face it. Most people who want to know more ask questions. People who don't may want, or need, to pretend it's not happening. In one study, about 15 percent of the cancer patients surveyed did not want to know about a fatal diagnosis.

It may well happen that a person tells us he or she is dying and that we must prepare ourselves. Dr. Kübler-Ross says, "Everyone knows when they're going to die, although it may be subconsciously."

If it comes to you to tell someone they may be dying, you can only do it in your own way. You might ask, "How sick are you?" If the answer is, "Well, I'm very sick...or dying," you might say, "Yes, that's my impression too." Remember, you're not telling them it's the end. It can be a time of satisfying new growth. You might suggest that a very sick person ask God what's happening instead of a doctor.

If someone asks you what's happening and you answer honestly and without killing hope, communication remains open for sharing thoughts and feelings. A person may know she or he is dying and ask you only for confirmation. If you aren't honest this time, the person may not trust you or feel free to share with you in the future.

BEING WITH SOMEONE WHO IS DYING

How can we most usefully be with someone who is dying? Just by being present with an open heart, making space for what is happening.

An open heart is love without conditions and judgments. Not, "I love you if..." just "I love you." No one is right or wrong. Fear, pain, and suffering are not right or wrong. Dying is not good or bad. Everything just is. From an open heart we can see all the needs of the person preparing for his or her great change.

To me, "serving humanity" is recognizing our common divinity. It doesn't necessarily mean being out there making the world over. Two people in a quiet bedroom can serve humanity. We serve just by understanding that we're both individual expressions of the One. We're not right or "up" because we're still healthy, and they are not wrong or "down" because they're sick and closer to dying. We are just two people surrendering to life, to all the things we may have thought life was about and have discovered it isn't. And the challenge is, can we keep our heart open to another's pain and sadness without closing it and shutting off our own pain? All pain is everyone's. Can we be open to what the dying can teach us about life?

We serve by recognizing that dying is okay. If we resist a person's dying, we may increase their resistance. If we pretend circumstances are different from what they are—deny what's happening—the dying have to play a painful charade with us. Pretending and not communicating isolate people from one another and make dying very lonely for everyone involved. Pretending can leave you both with the I-wish-I-hads: "I wish I'd said..." "I wish I'd done ..." Instead, we can do and say what we deeply feel. We can be open to the process of dying.

Our work is to make a supportive space to let someone die in their own way: to let the dying person be where she or he is, not to try to push them to where we'd like them to be. Dying with dignity is not necessarily dying with peace and acceptance, but dying in character.

Discuss all decisions relating to the dying person with him or her; even making decisions about small things allows a person to maintain their sense of dignity and worth. Help people express their preferences. If someone is accustomed to saying yes to things she or he doesn't like or want to do, encourage them to say no to those things. You might want to practice this yourself. Rather than overprotect them, encourage a dying person to live each day fully. In the face of death, does it matter if someone dies a little sooner because he or she went fishing or to a concert or enjoyed a binge on lobster, chili, or chocolate ice cream? We've nothing to lose that we won't lose anyway.

Don't assume you know how someone feels—ask. Don't force someone to eat or smile or be social. Those may be your needs, not his or hers. Try to be sensitive to the dying person's need to be with people or to be alone. Ask, "Is there anything else I can do for you?" This may uncover a need you couldn't have dreamed of. Once when I asked my dad, he answered, "Just don't stop loving me or helping me like you are."

Albert Schweitzer said, "There is a modesty of soul which we must recognize, just as we do that of the body. The soul, too, has its clothing of which we must not deprive it, and no one has the right to say to another, because we belong to each other, as we do, 'I have a right to know all of your thoughts.'"

Conditioned by our cultural fear of death, people expect a lot of difficult emotional and psychological problems around dying. In working with dying people and their families from many different backgrounds, I have seen few challenges the family couldn't handle. Those few I did witness were related to guilt, which occurs less often at home than in a hospital setting.

Don't sit around fearing problems that may never manifest. Here are some reassuring words from Dr. Sylvia A. Lack:

> *There is far too much talk in death and dying circles in this country about psychological and emotional problems, and far too little about making the patient comfortable. Any group concerned with service to the dying should be talking about smoothing sheets, rubbing bottoms, relieving constipation, and sitting up at night. Counseling a person who is lying in a wet*

bed is ineffective... If people are cared for with common sense and basic professional skills, with detailed attention to self-evident problems and physical needs, the patients and families themselves cope with many of their emotional crises. Without pain, well nursed, with bowels controlled, mouth clean, and a caring friend available, the psychological problems fall into manageable perspective.[1]

This is not to say challenges won't arise, just that you will be able to handle them.

Polite conventions and courteous fictions that people have maintained all their lives may drop away when they're dying. Old prejudices, resentments, and grievances may surface; long-hidden preferences (as for one child over another) may no longer be glossed over.

There may be conflict between family members or between family members and caregivers. Conflict is not "bad." It's an opportunity to clarify values. Two people (or countries) may be in conflict because they each care deeply about something, feel the other doesn't understand their feelings or respect their beliefs, and believe they're "right." Resolving conflict involves appreciating the other's belief, eliminating the judgments "right" and "wrong," and accepting that we differ and it's all right.

The dying person may pass through periods of generalized hostility toward everyone. If you are the object of this kind of projection, know that *it doesn't matter.* You are who you are, not who someone else *wants* you to be or *imagines* you to be. Someone may insult an image they have of you, but that is not you. You are not someone's reaction to you. Instead of reacting to the reaction, you can choose compassion and try to look deeper, to the person's essence. Mother Teresa calls it "touching Christ in his distressing disguise." We don't have to like someone's personality just because they're dying. We can always love who they really are.

We also serve by respecting our own needs. With the discomforts of dying, a sick person may become demanding. If you feel overwhelmed by their demands, tell them. We don't win prizes for being martyrs. If a person is acting irrational, don't be afraid to be firm. Again, look deeper to see what unspoken need is being expressed and try to meet it. There's no need to be over-polite. If the dying person is afraid to ask for something, and family members are afraid to do what comes naturally for fear of seeming pushy or hurting others' feelings, no one will be happy.

Jealousy—feeling someone has something you don't—may come up. This is natural. Someone other than you may appear to be the special one. Look inside yourself: how much more special can you be? You were born with your specialness. There will always be people who can see it and people who can't.

A dying person can also be a joy to be with. Take a moment before you enter their room to breathe in calmness: "Soften. Relax. Open." Be as natural as possible. Here is time you may not have made before for the quiet joy of sharing as a family, couple, or friends. The illusion of time—that there are things to do, places to go—can drop away: there are just moments for whatever is! Share your feelings and what's happening in your life. Ask the dying person's advice. His or her perspective from dying may be of great help to you.

When the person seems open, talk about what's happening, what they want done when they die, a will, what kind of burial...Often people feel more like talking in the evening or at night. Listen and listen. If there are things you've wanted to say or talk about with them and haven't, use this opportunity. It will ease your grieving later.

People who are sleeping or appear to be unconscious can still hear you at some level. Say only what you would say if they were totally awake. People confined to bed pick up the "vibrations" around them, perhaps more so than a physically active person who has more distractions.

Something I do each time before entering the room of a dying person may be of use to you. I say a prayer: "God, use me for whatever this person needs if that serves the highest good of us both." Then I share my heart, sometimes with words or just with my eyes and hands.

It is a rare privilege to be with someone who is dying. I suggest you use this time to think about your own death, your own spiritual beliefs. As we accept someone else's dying, we move toward accepting our own. See what you can learn from this dying that's useful for your life. What is really meaningful in your life, and what is it time to let go of? What do you want to be or do or say that you haven't? Make the most of the inevitable by *living fully* each moment and letting go of any sense of separateness.

If you find yourself working on two levels, one which says "dying is okay" and one which says "his or her dying is not okay," be gentle with yourself. The two will come together. There's an old circus adage that "you can't learn balance until you've learned to lose it."

Trust yourself. Love yourself.

THE DYING PERSON'S BILL OF RIGHTS[2]

This bill, created by the Southwestern Michigan In-service Education Council, shares the concerns of many dying people. Perhaps most importantly, it points toward the dyings' desire to choose what they do and don't want. For example, not all people want to die with someone present, but most want to make the choice.

I have the right to be treated as a living human being until I die.

I have the right to maintain a sense of hopefulness, however changing its focus may be.
I have the right to be cared for by those who can maintain a sense of hopefulness, however changing this might be.
I have the right to express my feelings and emotions about my approaching death, in my own way.
I have the right to participate in decisions concerning my care.
I have the right to expect continuing medical and nursing attention, even though "cure" goals must be changed to "comfort" goals.
I have the right not to die alone.
I have the right to be free of pain.
I have the right to have any questions answered honestly.
I have the right not to be deceived.
I have the right to have help from and for my family in accepting my death.
I have the right to die in peace and dignity.
I have the right to retain my individuality and not be judged for my decisions, which may be contrary to the beliefs of others.
I have the right to discuss and enlarge my religious and/or spiritual experiences, regardless of what they may mean to others.
I have the right to expect that the sanctity of the human body will be respected after death.
I have the right to be cared for by caring, sensitive, knowledgeable people who will attempt to understand my needs and will be able to gain some satisfaction in helping me face death.

THE SEARCH FOR MEANING

From the beginning of time until now, human beings have searched for meaning. Meaning gives us a reason to live, the courage to meet life's constant changes. We even tolerate pain if we can find meaning in it. If we've not done so earlier, as we die, we ponder the meaning of our lives.

In hospitals, dying people often lose their sense of life as meaningful. They lose hope, and when they lose hope, they die.

One of the great blessings of dying at home is that we're still surrounded by people and things that give immediate meaning to our lives as we search for ultimate meanings. Even at home, a dying person may go through periods of finding life meaningless and his or her present suffering hard to bear.

We can't find meaning for others, but we can share ideas that may point them toward discovering new meaning for them. Before talking with someone about meaning, be sure they're comfortable and free from pain. Share what is true for you as a gentle gift, not as dogma that makes the dying person "wrong" if he or she feels differently.

When someone is dying, many outside sources of meaning such as work and daily activities are no longer available. But instead of diminishing the meaning of life, surprisingly, dying people find life, just being alive, increasingly meaningful. With fewer outer distractions, they tend to look inward for the source of meaning. For many this is an unaccustomed place to look.

Looking inward, they find that the very fact of being alive has meaning—that meaning is not necessarily related to what we are able or not able to do. Life is recognized as precious and meaningful in and of itself, even if the trimmings are limited. Life is meaningful because it "is." It doesn't have to perform, show off, or justify itself.

To live fully, even in the face of death, is to live now in this moment. Only in the now of this moment can we experience the wholeness and holiness of life.

To help people find meaning in their lives is to help them live in the moment. Encourage them not to limit themselves to their pasts or their future, but to experience the unlimited now. For many this is difficult. We're accustomed to living off our memories of the past or our projections on the future.

Help the person you're caring for appreciate the preciousness of life, moment by moment. For in these moments, he or she will find meaning and peace and joy.

If it's appropriate for you, help them to appreciate the gift of receiving. Sometimes we forget the circle of love includes giving and receiving. For people who place great value on control or who don't often allow themselves to receive, accepting all the care a dying person needs is difficult. Needing and receiving make them feel helpless, worthless.

Many of us are graceful givers. Not so many of us are graceful receivers. We prefer giving because we've been praised for it since we were toddlers and because when we're giving, we're *in control.* We haven't usually been praised for receiving. Often receiving was labeled "selfish." We're afraid of receiving because when we're receiving, we're *vulnerable,* and that's scary. Perhaps we also doubt we're worthy of receiving or fear feeling indebted to the giver.

Help the dying understand that receiving is just as valuable and sacred as giving. Using your own words, help them understand the arrogance of always having to be the giver and denying others the joy of giving. Let them know that we help others to feel strong by allowing them to help us. You might perhaps remind a parent that they cared for all your needs for many years, and you're grateful now to have a chance to return that caring.

Help the dying understand the importance of balancing *doing* and *being.*

Our culture rewards us for *doing*—for achieving success, controlling nature, remaining young, and thinking rationally. It's not often that we get pats for just *being*—sitting quietly watching a stream, communing with God, listening to a child, being angry or old, crying or dying. We tend to forget the value of being: just being present for ourselves, for our feelings, or the child, stream, or dying person in front of us. We rush from one activity to another and then we're surprised when life feels meaningless, as if we've lost touch with something precious.

We've measured our lives by what we do. But life doesn't limit herself to doing. She includes being. Being present for our dying is just as valuable as any project or task well done. Perhaps it's the most courageous thing we will ever do.

By helping the dying understand that being is as important as doing, we help them adjust to not being able to do all the things they're accustomed to doing. If we primarily value doing, we can't accept death or find meaning in dying, and we can't help the dying do the same. Dying is a return to our original nature, to being.

Help the dying to understand that the most important thing a human being can do, they can continue to do: love. No illness, no prediction of limited days, can stop us from loving. Is there a greater meaning for a human life than love—to love and to allow ourselves to be loved?

When Mom was dying and feeling discouraged about all the things she could no longer do, I'd ask her, "Mom, what's the most important thing a human being can do?" She'd answer, "Love." My reply was, "Well then, you're still in great shape!"

Help the dying to enjoy the harvest of their lives, to remember their storehouse of love and joy. Talk together about the things you've shared together as a family, as friends. Death cannot take away our memories. Memory exists far beyond the gates of death.

Help the dying understand that life is lived most graciously when control and surrender are balanced. Often we humans believe that we must be in control of our lives, and that only if we are in control, are we truly living. We forget that surrender, accepting life as it is, is just as important.

Help the dying understand that they don't have to hold up life. They can let go and let life hold them up instead. To control is to do our will. To surrender is to let Life's will be done. Perhaps the underlying truth is that our will and Life's will are One.

If a dying person's religious beliefs give him or her a sense of meaning, support their understanding. Encourage them to explore their own teaching even more deeply—to move beyond dogma to the core of that particular teaching. The core of all religions is the same: love God, love yourself, love your fellow human beings, and know that we are one.

Again, take time as you care for this dying person to consider what's meaningful for you. The day of your death will come. And the more moments you have lived in alignment with what's meaningful to you, the more joyful your life will be and the easier will be your dying and death.

GRIEVING

Like a bird singing in the rain,
Let grateful memories survive in time of sorrow.

—Robert Louis Stevenson

Grieving is opening up to sadness or anger if we feel it, and releasing it. We need to grieve throughout this dying-loving process to keep cleansing and clearing ourselves. If we don't, we're liable to walk through the whole experience numb from the strain of holding our feelings in. When we become so full of sadness that we can't hold any more, we close our hearts. If we wait until "it's all over" to open the floodgates, the backed-up emotion may seem overwhelming.

The gift of grieving is that it allows us to open to the reservoir of sadness in each of us, much of it not even related to the dying process we're living now. Grieving is an opportunity to clean up old, old stuff—the attic or basement of our beings so we can move ahead with greater lightness, space, and freedom.

Let the person you're supporting, man or woman, know that crying is a way to cleanse ourselves so we can live more fully. Cry as much as you need to give yourself more space for living.

Chapter 15 addresses the grief you may experience after the death.

PACING YOURSELF, FAMILY HEALTH, AND MORALE

Let there be spaces in your togetherness,
and let the winds of the heavens dance between you.

—Kahlil Gibran
Mystic and author of *The Prophet*

Time is often the great unknown factor in a dying process. Unlike a home birth, in which the baby is born within a relatively short time, a dying process has no fixed time limit. Not knowing "how long we have" is hard for the dying person and the family. For this reason, pacing yourself is very important.

Nobody can face death all the time, neither the sick person nor the family. Unless you take time for yourself, for letting out your feelings and taking care of your health, you may well run out of fuel before the process is over. An early all-out effort can exhaust you and cause you to resent the dying person for taking so much of your time and energy. Contrary to all beliefs and appearances, you are not Superman or Wonder Woman, although a part of you may think you should be.

Before you get out of bed each day, you might want to ask yourself, "What nice thing can I do for myself today?" This might become a morning meditation to give yourself more energy for the day. Meditation is not some mysterious Hindu or Buddhist practice. It means living with awareness. Being aware the toast is burning, being aware of God. To some people, meditation is something done in a time or place specially set aside for this purpose. But, all of life can be a meditation.

Because you're probably spending more time at home than usual, do some things you've wanted to do at home and haven't. Pick flowers. Make a fresh juice cocktail. Take a walk. Write a letter. When Mary was with me, I did a lot of sewing and caught up on paperwork. Instead of thinking, "God, I'm getting behind," I could think, "Great! I'm getting stuff done I wouldn't if I weren't home so much." While my dad was dying, I continued to work on the first edition of this book.

Exercise, eat well, and get as much sleep as possible. Try to eat balanced meals and not live on coffee and doughnuts. Taking Vitamin B and/or brewer's yeast may help soothe your nerves and give you energy. If possible, keep your own bedroom. With Mary, I was comforted to have my own space and sleep in my own bedroom but still be able to hear her if I kept the door open. If someone needs constant attention, you'll need people with whom you can rotate sleeping. If you have no help, you may have to sleep in the room with the dying person, and you may want to anyway.

Taking care of family morale includes doing enjoyable things for yourself as well as with the dying person. Don't be afraid to ask for help so you can go out or have time alone. Go to the movies, dancing, bowling, or to a botanical garden or a restaurant you've wanted to try. Visit with friends and talk about it all. You can be totally loving and not think about the dying person all the time. Ask for help if you need someone simply to be with you. By asking, you give someone else a chance to share love. If they don't respond as you hope, respect their honesty. Perhaps they'll volunteer on another occasion.

If there are children in the family, include them in what's happening and make time to focus on their needs as well as the dying person's (see chapter 8.).

If you are participating in a hospice program, remember that respite care is included. Respite care provides five days in a residential hospice, nursing home, or hospital for your loved one, so that you can take time to rest up at home, attend a special event, or take a mini vacation. There is no limit to the number of five-day periods you can take. You pay 5 percent of what Medicare pays per day for the dying person's care. For example, if Medicare has to pay $100 per day for their care, you pay $5.

Please ask for help when you need it. Be kind enough to yourself to recognize when you've hit your limits. Medical professionals now recognize what they call caregiver syndrome: mental and physical illnesses rooted in stress, exhaustion, and self-neglect. If you find yourself feeling angry or frustrated, a part of you is calling out for help. Skip the guilt.

At one time in my journey with Mom, I brought her to Hawaii where I cared for her full time with a few hours' break three days a week. After a while, I began falling apart physically and emotionally because I couldn't get the sleep I needed. One day as I was helping her down the stairs to her wheelchair at the bottom, I thought, "If I pushed her, I could sleep tonight." Shocked that such a morbid thought could even cross my mind, I finally realized I was in over my head and needed help. Within a week, we returned to Texas and a nursing home.

Even if it's very difficult, honor yourself as well as your loved one. Skip guilt. You're just as important as the dying person.

If you run "caregiver" through an online search engine, you will find a multitude of sites with useful information (see appendix C).

SHARING

Sharing with a dying person lets them know they still count. While you're emotionally letting them go, it's important for you to be conscious that they're not gone until they're gone.

What can you share? Share your feelings as it feels appropriate, but not to the point of burdening the dying person. It may be hard the first time, but it gets easier.

Share time together. Share decisions. Share games. Are there TV programs or stories you can enjoy together? Read together. Remember good times together. Pray together.

Another idea is to ask yourself each morning, "What nice thing can we do as a family or group of friends today?"

What about asking the dying person to share the story of his or her life or making a tape recording (as we did with my dad) or a video? These memories may help the dying person understand the tapestry of his or her life, and be a source of joy and comfort to you.

An organization called Story Corps, dedicated to recording ordinary peoples' stories and archiving them in the Library of Congress, published a book entitled *Listening Is an Act of Love.* The following are some starter questions:

- What is the most important lesson you have learned in life?
- What are you proud of?
- Do you have any regrets?

- What was the happiest moment of your life?
- The saddest?
- How would you like to be remembered?

Anybody like to play Scrabble? Here are two other games that may be fun to play with someone in bed whose mind is clear.

Dictionary Game: For four or more players. You'll need a dictionary, paper, and pencils. One person (the starter) goes first and chooses a word from the dictionary whose meaning she or he doesn't think any other player knows. It can't be a word starting with a capital letter. The starter reads only the word and then writes down the dictionary definition in his or her own words. Each player writes a definition that seems right or invents one that's amusing. Then everyone passes in his or her definition to the starter, who reads all of them, not distinguishing between the dictionary definition and the rest (which means reading over them first in case someone's writing isn't clear). Everyone then guesses which is the correct definition. Then the starter reads the dictionary definition.

A player gets ten points for writing the dictionary definition and five points if he or she guesses one someone else wrote. Play until you're tired of playing and add up the points—if anyone cares. In my family we didn't often bother to keep score. We just played for the laughs.

Analogy: For as many players as you want. One person (the starter) secretly picks a person in the room. If there aren't many of you, include someone whom everyone knows. Each player uses an analogy to obtain clues about who this person is. The object, obviously, is to name the person. The player asks, "If she or he were a bird, what kind of bird would she or he be?" "If she or he were a flower, instrument, cloud, car...?" The starter answers with the analogy: "She'd be a seagull or a pelican." As soon as you have a feeling about who it might be, guess!

VISITORS

Put yourself in the dying person's shoes and realize–
truly realize in your heart, not just in your intellect–
that one day you could be, more than likely will be,
in the same situation.

—Peter Weatherby
The Pilgrim Soul

The number of friends a dying person wants to see usually depends on his or her earlier lifestyle. People who enjoy having lots of people around will probably continue to do so. Someone more solitary will probably want to see only a few. Ask if the person wants visitors. Ask if it's okay for someone to bring along a child.

Visits with a dying person are usually short, unless the person indicates otherwise. Visits can take a lot of energy, and some people feel drained afterward. If, as a visitor, you're open to your own feelings, including sadness, your visit will likely give energy instead of take it. Ask the dying person if he or she is tired, and perhaps the visit should end. If some of you want to visit longer, move to another room.

Let visitors know what mood the person seems to be in today. If they haven't seen their friend in a long time, let them know how she or he looks now. It softens the shock if visitors know, for example, that their old robust 180-pound friend is down to 100 pounds.

If the dying person has expressed a wish not to see someone, respect this wish. I advise not sending anyone into the room who is extremely upset or negative. You might first help such a visitor express his or her feelings with you. Then, if they have a real need to see the person, accompany them and stand by for the "enough" signal from the patient. At the same time, don't overprotect. The dying person and visitor may need to be alone to sort out a misunderstanding, and they might both feel better afterward.

As a visitor, be sensitive to your friend, to what is appropriate to share with him or her now. Imagine what it feels like if someone says, "You look great!" or "Let's go fishing next spring." How would you feel if you received a "get well" card and you knew you weren't going to get well? These are obvious clues to a dying person that someone can't handle their dying, which makes real communication impossible. The dying person usually agrees to play along and pretend the illness is temporary, and after the visitor leaves, he or she is probably left feeling quite alone.

If business considerations need to be discussed, first check with the family to find out when it might be appropriate.

Instead of making general offers, like "Call me if you need anything," make a specific offer: "I'll bring dinner tomorrow night" or "I'll take the kids to the zoo Saturday."

As people approach death, they need more and more time alone to prepare for the transition. Don't take it personally if the sick person doesn't want to see you or doesn't recognize you. This is not uncommon. There's no need to feel badly. Focusing inward and disconnecting from the outer world is a natural part of the dying process.

If you'd like to know more about ways to help, I recommend an excellent pamphlet called *Is There Anything I Can Do to Help,* published by Medic Publishing Company. If I feel anxious, reading *Emanuel's Book,* by Pat Rodegast, helps me to remember the bigger picture, relax, and sleep well. I highly recommend it.

To support your sharing with friends and family who may be distant, I also recommend creating a free web site with Caring Bridges, a nonprofit organization. It's easy to do, even for a non-techy, and it provides you with a place to post what is happening with you and your loved one and where friends and family can respond. This may perhaps save you fielding more phone calls than you want to handle at this time yet allow you to maintain relationships that you treasure.

TO ALL PARENTS

"I'll lend you for a little time
a child of Mine," He said,
"For you to love the while he lives,
and mourn for when he's dead.
It may be six or seven years,
or twenty-two or -three,
But will you, 'til I call him back,
take care of him for me?
He'll bring his charms to gladden you
and shall his stay be brief
You'll bring his lovely memories
as solace for your grief.

I cannot promise he will stay
since all from earth return,
But there are lessons taught down there
I want this child to learn.
I've looked the wide world over,
in My search for teachers true
And from the throngs that crowd life's lanes,
I have selected you.
Now, will you give him all your love,
not think the labor vain,
Nor hate Me when I come to call
to take him back again?

I fancied that I heard you say,
"Dear Lord Thy Will be done.
For all the joy Thy child shall bring,
the risk of grief we'll run.
We'll shelter him with tenderness;
We'll love him while we may
And for the happiness we've known,
Forever grateful stay;
But shall the angels call for him
much sooner than we've planned
We'll brave the painful grief that comes
and try to understand."

—Edgar A. Guest

8

CHILDREN

Mama, can we still laugh?

—A child's question about dying

CHILDREN AS MEMBERS OF THE FAMILY

Allowing a child to participate at home in the death of someone she or he loves can be an incredible gift. Children can learn early that death is a natural part of life. Without automatically acquiring our culture's fear, a child chooses his or her own attitude about death.

When a dying family member is isolated in a hospital, often with "no visitors under thirteen," the child has no way of developing a healthy attitude. Even if our words say "Death is okay," the child feels left out, wondering what's going on and scared because he or she can't see or share in what's happening.

Shielding children from death makes them fear it more and makes it more difficult to accept death as adults. Shielding children from our feelings when someone we love is dying teaches them to deny their feelings, which closes their hearts. Out of love, we have tried to protect them. Out of love, let us free them instead.

The loss of someone a child loves is more bearable if she or he has shared in the dying process. The shock is less if the child has time to adjust *gradually* to the loss. Being at home together allows this gradual adjustment, as well as time for what can be a very beautiful sharing.

A child's greatest fear is separation from or loss of a parent. At home together, parents can help the child understand that in our hearts we never lose anyone. We feel very sad someone won't be with us and we can feel joy for the love we'll always share.

For many of us, talking with our children about death ranks second in uncomfortableness only to the "birds and bees" conversation. And it's our responsibility to talk about death clearly and truthfully when it comes up. Helping children relate to the deaths of birds and animals offers an opportunity to help them develop a healthy acceptance of death. Don't discourage children from touching dead creatures. They can always wash their hands and it helps them to understand.

What a child imagines about dying may be worse than the truth. Euphemisms and white lies mislead and confuse a child about what's happening. If you say that someone who died has "just gone to sleep," your child may be afraid to go to bed. If you say, "God took him," your child may spend his life fearing or hating God.

One way of explaining death is to say, "Jimmie was too sick to get well and he stopped breathing." *Immediately reassure* the child that she or he will get well from flu or a cold, or any familiar sickness. Then go on to explain your spiritual beliefs. A friend's little boy, after the death of his brother asked, "Where is Damian?" His mother replied, "Always in your heart." She said his acceptance was happy and instantaneous.

Explain death in your own way. Use words or ideas a child can understand. Share facts (not too technical) as well as your feelings. Allow space for your child to develop his or her own understanding of death by admitting you don't know everything. Ask your child what he or she thinks. Be patient if children bring up the subject of death again and again as they try to understand it.

Children are often afraid of the dark and of being alone. What they fear for themselves, they often fear for the dying person. It seems honest to reassure them, based on near-death experiences, that there will be beautiful light, love, and loving people to meet the dying person (see chapter 16).

When we talk with children about dying, it's important that we share our sadness as well as the reassurance that the dying person is going to a beautiful place. This helps them understand the seeming contradiction between our words and our behavior. Elisabeth Kübler-Ross said we say, "Mommy is going to heaven," because it's true! But when nobody's celebrating, our children won't believe us unless we share our personal loss as well.

Unless we've helped our children understand in some way that there's life apart from the physical body, they won't believe Mommy is going to a beautiful place when they see her put in a hole in the earth. These days, in our materialistic world, *soul* is not a particularly fashionable word. Perhaps it needs reinstating because it's useful to have a name for the consciousness apart from the body that never dies. You might explain *soul* to children using the metaphor of the cocoon and the butterfly: we leave the old shell to become something even more beautiful.

What children need most when someone they love is dying is reassurance. Reassure them that they're loved and will be cared for. Reassure them that they're safe and aren't likely to die for a long time. Reassure them that besides the absence of the dying person, their world will stay more or less the same. Reassure them that the death is not their fault. Children tend to take responsibility for everything that happens in their little worlds. Often they feel guilty when someone they love is dying: "It's my fault because I was bad."

Often when someone we love is dying, we become totally preoccupied with that person, particularly if it's a dying child. Remember to keep the circle of love open to the whole family.

If you have more than one child, spend time alone with each. A crying child and a less demonstrative one both need attention. Tears are not the only measure of grief.

Include your children in what's happening. Children feel good about sharing the responsibility of making the dying person comfortable. They feel important to be included in this family event. Let them participate in any way they want. Ask for their help with tasks they can handle. Hugging, holding, and cuddling are some of our best medicines, and children are experts in delivering them.

Children can provide comfort and welcome relief from the intensity of dying. Including them can also prevent having to deal later with a demanding or uncommunicative child who feels unloved, rejected, and/or guilty. You don't have to do anything special for them; they understand Mom doesn't have time to take them to the zoo or whatever activities they enjoy together. Just include them.

Children usually adjust easily to being around a dying adult or child if they're told what's happening and are included. They adjust more easily than adults if they haven't been overly conditioned to think death is terrible. Don't *banish* the kids to Grandma's or Auntie's. It's likely to increase their fears. Do *send* them if you need a break. Children can feel the difference.

Sometimes we shower attention and gifts on a dying child and forget our other children may feel jealous. It's common for children to feel jealous, to wish a dying brother or sister who's getting all the attention were dead, and then to feel guilty for those feelings. It might be helpful to say to a child you suspect feels this way something like, "I would understand if you're angry because I spend so much time with Annie...or if you sometimes wish she were already dead. You know, we just have a short time with her, and you and I will probably have our whole lives together."

Remember not to make a dying child seem perfect in every way. It's too high a standard for our other children to live up to.

Include your children in the family's grief. Let them see you grieving instead of trying to hide it. This provides a healthy model for accepting and healing their pain now and in the future. Children shielded from your feelings may feel rejected. It may be distressing to see Dad cry, but "business as usual" is more distressing. Wildly excessive expression of grief, however, may not be wholesome and may cause a child to fear their feelings.

Encourage children to express their feelings, fears, and fantasies. Let them know it's okay to cry—"Big, strong people cry sometimes"—and it's okay to be angry. They may be angry because you can't prevent the death. They often feel angry that they're being abandoned. Don't put unnecessary burdens on children by saying things like "Be brave" or "Now you'll be the man of the house" or "You have to take care of Daddy."

Help your children keep up with other relationships and continue to have friends in to play. Watching children play quietly may delight the dying person; if not, ask them to play in another room. Ben and Josh were a big help to us in terms of joy, humor, entertainment, and keeping life in perspective.

Help your children express their feelings by encouraging them to say whatever they want to the dying person. Encourage drawing and telling stories. Stories children tell that don't correspond with an adult's reality are not necessarily lies. They're children's ways of sharing their reality, which can help us understand how to better support them.

If you have school-age children, let their teachers and school counselor know someone in the family is dying. They're usually glad to give extra support. Don't be concerned if children are distracted from school work and their grades drop. They go through the process of grieving too. If they want to stay home from school and help, consider occasionally letting them do so. A very special school is happening in your own home.

Some children's books I love that focus on death and dying are Ethel Marback's *The Cabbage Moth and the Shamrock* (Green Tiger Press), Flynn's *Mister God, This is Anna* (Ballantine Books) for older children and adults, and Leo Buscaglia's *The Fall of Freddie the Leaf.*

TO PARENTS OF DYING CHILDREN

Mamma, Papa, don't be afraid.

—A dying child

Your child will give you the support you need.

—A mother whose child died at home

I have not yet worked with children dying at home. I have worked with parents of dying children and parents grieving after the death.

For most of us, accepting a child dying is much harder than accepting an adult dying. For a mother and father, it may be the hardest thing they ever face. And there's no preparation other than living and loving fully each moment and holding our children lightly, knowing they are just on loan.

There are no words that will take away your pain if your child is dying. There are, however, some ideas that may help prevent bitterness or resentment.

We may feel bitter because a child has "everything to look forward to," "their whole life ahead of them." We experience time as linear and sequential and feel a child who dies young was incomplete, cut off before their time.

Perhaps it would help to remember that a child is complete and whole at each moment in the process of his or her life. Our vision might be more like the Native American vision. The original Americans understood time as an "expanded present."

In a 1998 article in *Omni Magazine* entitled "The American Indian Mind," Barry Lopez wrote the following:

Most Native Americans did not understand their lives as a sequence of goals (getting an education, getting married, raising children, being an elder) at the end of which lay a sense of final completion. For them, once one entered adulthood, often at the age of only ten or twelve, life was complete. One could only continue to grow in that state—in the way a sphere, already complete, can continue to expand, to become fuller. There was no thought of not having done enough in one's life, of being too young to die, or of still having your whole life ahead of you.

With that continuous sense of a full life, no one was tyrannized by the prospect of death. Any day, but especially one in which you were living to the hilt, was a good day to die.[1]

I believe it's accurate to enlarge that understanding to include all ages.

Everyone is complete at every moment.

When a child is dying, we often ask ourselves why—a question for which we may not find a satisfactory answer. I encourage you instead to ask, "What can I learn?" "What have I learned from my child?" Even now, if you're willing, close your eyes for a moment and think and feel about what you've learned. Among your answers, I imagine, will be love—unconditional love—and joy.

I ask you from "our" heart, "Is there a greater purpose for a human life than to be a teacher of love and joy? Are going to school, growing up, getting a job, getting married, and growing old more important?"

Besides coming to gain experience to be fully who they can be, perhaps each child comes to teach us unconditional love—that quality that allows us to experience the sacredness of life. Your life and my life are sacred. Perhaps children who come for only a short time come to remind us not to take anyone or anything for granted, that every moment of life is a precious gift. I believe there's no such thing as a "child," only wise old souls in children's bodies.

Even as you grieve for an incredible loss, as your heart breaks open, celebrate love.

I believe there is so much love in each of us that we create a child partially as a place to put that love. Often we give all our love to our child and forget to love ourselves. Then, if he or she is dying, we feel like love is dying as well. Perhaps a child dies to give us an opportunity to remember that we are love. One mother, after her boy died, said, "He made me see the love inside myself."

The physical loss of your child is a great sadness that must be grieved for. It is not the loss of your love. Love is the very nature of your being. It doesn't die, even when the object of your love changes form. It is redistributed. Do not burden your child with responsibility for your love or burden yourself with fear of its loss. That is more than either of you needs to bear.

The pain we feel when a child is dying comes not only from believing love dies, but also from holding on. No one can tell you how or when to let go, to surrender. The moment of acceptance comes in its own time and way. Perhaps it's useful to remember the child was never really "yours" to begin with. She or he always belonged to Life, to God.

Pain can also come from expecting ourselves to be perfect parents. We pooh-pooh the idea of being perfect ones, yet we secretly expect ourselves to be. Often we feel angry and guilty when we can't prevent our child's death. You could not prevent your child's death any more than you could prevent a river from flowing to the sea.

Forgive yourself for being so hard on yourself. Forgive yourself for all the things you did or said that you now regret. Forgive yourself for all the things you didn't do or say that you think you should have. Forgive your child for dying.

You will survive this experience. You will survive. Life goes on even if you've forgotten quite why.

Even as survival dominates your consciousness, hold the seed of hope. You feel love even as you grieve, and you can feel joy again if you'll let yourself. Some parents won't. They feel it would somehow be disloyal to their child—a sign they didn't really love them. Others have allowed joy again—perhaps a more fitting tribute to a child, to a teacher of love, than suffering.

I've asked many parents what they learned from their child's death. I still remember the radiant faces of two mothers, one of whom had two children die, as they answered, "Joy." They weren't joyful that their children died. They had learned from them that life is precious, love is all that really matters, and each moment is best lived fully because we don't know how many moments we have. A life lived from these understandings is a joyful life.

Unfortunately, we live in a culture that often measures love by suffering. Suffering is proof of how much we love. We expect parents of children who have died to wear invisible scarlet letters over their hearts. We expect them to be "scarred for life."

I regularly hear grieving parents and professional caregivers say to other grieving parents, "You never get over it,"

"You'll never stop grieving," "You'll never be the same." With good intentions, they condemn parents to a lifetime of pain. When someone hurts more than they've ever hurt, telling them it won't stop is like kicking them in the gut when they're already down. It makes me mad. And it's not true, unless you believe them and make it come true. Many parents do stop grieving and return to living fully without the haunting shadow of pain.

What you never stop is loving and remembering your child. True, you'll never be the same, but that doesn't have to be negative. It may be a blessing.

At the same time we expect parents not to stop grieving, we also expect them to act as if nothing happened. Sometimes this short-circuits the grieving process and the result is self-pity. There's nothing wrong with feeling sorry for ourselves. We all have. As they say, "It's easier for others to count our blessings." Self-pity, though, doesn't feel good, and there's an alternative: grieving.

Time does not heal. It just pushes things into the back of our consciousness. What heals is what we do with time; grieving heals. The way home to joy is through the heart of our pain. We have to grieve until we come out the other side of it.

You don't have to go into the heart of your pain alone... unless you want to. Your husband, wife, wise friend, or counselor can accompany you without interfering. If you want to be physically alone, or you are, walk into your heart with God, Christ, Buddha, Mohammed, or with whoever is meaningful to you.

The widow of the poet Dylan Thomas wrote a book with the saddest title I've ever heard: *Leftover Life to Kill.* Grieve now, dear mother and father, so you don't have leftover life to kill. An emotional wound needs the same priority attention as a physical wound. For ways to work with your feelings, see chapter 10.

A tragedy is a loss without meaning. *Tragedy* literally means, in Greek, "the song of the goat." Your child dying is a great loss; it doesn't have to be a tragedy. A tragedy would be to go through the ecstasy and agony of creating and releasing a child and not to learn what he or she came to teach you.

Celebrate your child even as you live through this experience. Use this opportunity to give love to yourself, to the child inside you. In case you've forgotten, you're as important as your dying child.

In your own way, honor the great gift of your child.

❧

The following was shared with me by a mother whose child died:

EBONY

At the age of 2–1/2 years, Ebony became very sick. For almost a year we lived at the hospital, going through endless tests, drugs, and tears trying to understand why her central nervous system was breaking down. We never did get any real answers as to what went wrong or why.

Three months prior to her dying, I was at the height of my grieving. I was so angry with God! But God was big enough to handle my anger, and helped me understand the wonderful healing that comes from death. A week before Ebony's death, I came to total acceptance of the purpose for her life and I was at peace.

During the last day of Ebony's earthly life, my husband I took turns holding her in our arms. I remember feeling exactly the same way I did when I was giving birth to her...the same pain. The dying was like going through labor again. Tears... and tears...I felt I could not take much more pain. When she died, it was like the crowning—such relief, such peace, such utter joy!

My child's body lay dead in my arms, and I was feeling total joy and peace. I knew this was the greatest healing for her. What more could I want for my child who had suffered so much the past year.

—Karen Rockwood

NOTES ON DYING CHILDREN

I'd like to share a few ideas I've encountered during my work with dying adults and parents whose children died.

According to parents and other caregivers who work with dying children, children generally die more easily than adults. They have less fear of death because they haven't been as conditioned as adults have to fear it. Perhaps they're less fearful because they're closer to their *source.*

Except in unusual circumstances, children are happier at home than in a hospital. Most fear going to the hospital. They're afraid of being separated from you, of being alone in unfamiliar places where unfamiliar things happen. Sometimes they don't tell us how they really feel because they're afraid we'll take them to the hospital. Once you've decided your child will die at home, let him or her know you'll stay home together if it's at all possible.

If a child must spend time in a hospital, I encourage you to be there as much as possible. Consider asking permission from the doctor to take turns sleeping in a bed beside him or her. This isn't always possible, and depending on the personality and age of the child, may not be advisable. Remember, your other children and your husband or wife also deserve your care.

Children, like adults, fear mutilation. Having your child practice giving shots or other necessary procedures on a stuffed animal may ease the fear. Consider putting a dying child's bed in the living room so he or she can live and be cared for in the middle of the family. There you can rest and cuddle or sleep together.

Kids generally want to be like other kids. Within the limits created by the illness, help them to do this. They don't want people to feel sorry for them. Let other children or adults know that.

Help them feel as happy and secure as possible by not overwhelming them with your grief. This doesn't mean not to share your sadness. Again, hugging and holding are great healers for you both.

Children, even three or four year olds, can talk about their death. It may be in a symbolic way. Encourage a child to draw pictures about what she or he is feeling. What the child draws in the upper left quadrant of the picture supposedly indicates his or her feelings about the future and dying. Encourage a child to talk about the drawing by asking, "What's that about?" If we deliberately guess wrong a few times about the meaning of something in the picture, often the child can hardly wait to blurt out his or her truth.

You might ask a dying child, "What do you think it would be like to die?" This could open a conversation that might alleviate some fear for both of you. It might be an opportunity to share your spiritual beliefs.

Encourage an older dying child to write a letter to you, the parents, or to brothers and sisters.

Have you told your child how much you've loved being his or her mother or father?

A DYING BOY'S LETTER TO DOCTORS AND NURSES

I am dying...No one likes to talk about such things. In fact, no one likes to talk about much at all...I am the one who is dying. I know you feel insecure, don't know what to say, don't know what to do. But please believe me, if you care you can't go wrong. Just admit that you care. This is all we search for. We may ask for whys and wherefores, but we really don't want answers. Don't run away. Wait. All I want to know is that there will be someone to hold my hand when I need it. I'm afraid...I've never died before.

—Ron Klingbeil
A thirteen-year-old who died of leukemia

MARRIAGE AND PARTNERSHIPS

Sticks and stone are hard on bones,
aimed with an angry art.
Words can sting like anything,
but silence breaks the heart.

—Anonymous

In the mornings I lay in bed, hiding under the sheets, hating my husband for having someplace to go, for getting away from home, for having work to lose himself in. I felt we should have been growing closer during our suffering, getting strength from one another, instead, we were miles apart, sustaining a quiet politeness, drinking too much and pretending in others' company that we were doing alright...Sometimes I feel like I need to wear a sandwich board which reads, "Don't push me. I may shatter."

—Nancy Whittington
A mother whose child died

One way to define marriage is as a commitment to embrace the ups and downs of life together, and you may already be aware that a dying child can put a severe strain on that commitment. After the death of a child, a marriage rarely stays the same. It usually gets better or worse. Divorce rates after a child's death are very high. To avoid becoming a divorce statistic will take work.

We like to imagine partners leaning on each other for support as they care for their dying child. Yet that's often not true. If both parents are overwhelmed with grief, neither is available to be leaned on.

Sometimes the relationship between a mother and a dying child is so intense that it excludes, to varying degrees, the father. A father has a different, and often unappreciated, set of circumstances than a mother when his child is dying.

Often a mother is able to stay home and devote her whole being to her child; the father feels compelled to continue working. At work he's expected to function normally, so he hides his pain. He comes home exhausted from the strain of functioning "normally" and holding in his pain. Then the mother expects him to express his feelings, and if he doesn't, she's angry because he doesn't care *enough.* Our culture hasn't taught him to express his feelings. He can't stuff them down one minute and pull them up the next. Whatever he does, he's "wrong."

Don't expect your partner to grieve in the same way you do. You're two different people, and you each have your own way of dealing with grief. Expecting your partner to respond your way is how you set yourself up to feel angry and/or resentful. Anger and resentment are our responses to unfulfilled expectations.

Keep communication open as best you can. Keeping it open might be simply saying, "I love you and I can't talk now. Let's talk after supper." Schedule time to be alone as a couple. I know that's difficult, but wouldn't it be worth it to preserve or improve your marriage? Often one partner is able to talk more easily about what's happening. A less-talkative partner can listen and may eventually talk too.

Don't harbor little grievances. Talk about them before they're a huge pile of ammunition. What's the unexpressed need underlying the grievance?

Blame is harmful to any relationship. It's devastating to a marriage when a child is dying or has died. A grieving partner can't handle accusations, spoken or unspoken, such as "It's your fault he got worse because..." or "It's your fault she died because..." Spare each other. You're both doing the best you know how.

Your sexual relationship may disintegrate when your child is dying. If, in time after the death, it doesn't return to normal, seek a counselor. Inability to relate sexually often points to a deeper lack of communication.

Financial worries caused by a long illness can strain a marriage. If you're in over your head financially, consider a debt counselor instead of taking your fear out on each other.

If your marriage is suffering because you're so locked into pain you can't nurture it, seeing a counselor or social worker skilled in grief counseling could help. Hospices have bereavement counselors, or groups such as Compassionate Friends can offer support. (See appendix C for contact information.) I highly recommend *Healing a Father's Grief,* a booklet published by Medic Publishing Company.

Love yourself and your partner. Take care of each other. Forgive each other. Respect your individual ways of grieving. Keep communication open. Your partner will be here when your child is not.

A way I like to define marriage is a commitment to move to the truth together. The truth is love. Your child is your teacher.

You are love. You come from love. You are made by love. You cannot cease to be love. The whole manifestation is the manifestation of love. God himself is love. So the love which comes from the source, returns to the Source—and the purpose of life is accomplished in this.

—Hazrat Inayat Khan
The Purpose of Life

9

MAKING THE SENSES COMFORTABLE: PRACTICAL HOME CARE

Nothing is worth doing unless it's done with joy.

—A deva
Dorothy Maclean
To Hear the Angels Sing

Caring for someone means making the senses of the body comfortable, as well as the feelings, mind, and soul. A joyful, loving attitude as we provide physical care helps a dying person maintain or regain comfort and dignity. If we feel someone is glad to help us, we feel free to ask for what we want and need. On the other hand, if we feel we're a burden or nuisance, we're often afraid to ask. You might let the person know, "I enjoyed giving you a backrub," or, "Helping you is a pleasure, Dad."

I hope you're beginning to sense that this adventure you've begun can be a beautiful experience and even a creative art that you develop in your own way to please your patient and yourself. True creation comes from joy. Can you imagine duty creating a flower? Let yourself really enjoy creating comfort and beauty.

Dying well is a concern as old as we humans. What has changed is the meaning of *well. Ars Moriendi* (Dying Arts), which taught the art of dying, was one of the world's first do-it-yourself books. In the fifteenth century, Caxton produced a book, *Art and Craft to Know ye Well to Dye,* which included instructions for everything from the art of blowing your nose to weeping well.

Part of making people feel comfortable is knowing what we're doing. I suggest tacking a schedule or list on the kitchen wall for anything you need to keep track of. The list could include times for medication, diet, or who's going to be with the person if several people share the caring. Stay flexible; a list is just an aid. Remember, one of the reasons for being at home is doing what the dying person wants or needs instead of what's convenient for a hospital staff.

TOUCH

Your daily life is your temple and your religion.

—Kahlil Gibran

Touch is a way to share the love and caring in our hearts. It's important to all of us in endless ways. By touching a dying person, we physically express that something beyond physicality is important. A person is loved even if his or her body is unpleasant to see.

In many slow deaths from cancer, the body may become very unattractive physically. You may feel repulsed. It's a natural feeling. Keep your heart open and remember your touch is received by the person who owns the body. John, Mary, and my father did not have beautiful bodies when they died, yet each was a person of great beauty. By touching a dying person freely and lovingly, we're saying, "I care about you. You're more to me than just a body." This helps people understand that their bodies are only a part of who they are and helps them prepare to let go.

Massage

Massage is a beautiful way to touch and make a person comfortable. It also helps prevent bedsores. Even if you've never given a massage before, you can do it.

You may massage the head, hands, feet, back, or whole body. Do what you have time for and feel comfortable with. I'm particularly fond of foot massages because sometimes I'm too tired to do a person's whole body. Hands and feet have nerve endings from all the organs in the body. By massaging them, you stimulate and relax the body.

To avoid loosening possible blood clots, skip massaging the legs of people who have had recent surgery, have been bedridden for a long time, or are elderly.

Here are some simple massage instructions:

1. Before you start, make sure the room is warm enough and uncover only the part of the body you're going to massage.
2. Think about your love for the person.
3. Feel your hands as an extension of your heart and rub them together to make sure they're warm.
4. Let go of rushing around. Focus completely on this person.
5. Quietly enter the rhythm of their breathing; align your breathing with theirs.
6. Gently place your hands on the person, knowing the flesh may be very tender.
7. Trust your hands. They may be uncertain at first, but soon your instincts will open to what feels good to both of you. Light, flowing strokes can be very soothing.
8. Don't be afraid to say, "Tell me what feels good and what doesn't."
9. If your hands feel heavy or cramped, gently take them off the person for a moment and shake them.

10. Pay particular attention to bony areas like the tailbone, shoulder blades, or sides of the knees. If they are white or reddened, use your fingertips and rub in small circles around them, not on them. This will increase the blood supply and help prevent bedsores.
11. When you're through, keep your hands quietly on the person for a moment, then lift them off very slowly and gently. (I say a little prayer to myself that God bless the person.) If you remove your hands abruptly, the person is likely to feel a little deserted and shocked, negating some of the good feelings of the massage.
12. Cover the person when you finish, and help them feel cozy. They may drift off into tranquil sleep or feel so secure and loved they want to talk about things unsaid before.
13. Wash your hands in cool water to clear energy you may have picked up.

You're probably feeling better now yourself.

Hugging, Holding, and Cuddling

They're a cure for loneliness and our illusion of separateness. As long as they come from unconditional love, I don't think we can over-hug or over-cuddle. Sharing love and warmth may include an adult person's sexuality. This is okay.

Don't be afraid to ask for a hug. Your asking gives people a splendid opportunity, and if they don't want to give or share one, they can always say no. What about calling a morning "hug time" for your family? It's a great way to start the day. Jog to a friend's house for a hug. I once started a "morning hug" for my construction crew. We were the happiest workers on the site.

Your hugging, holding, and cuddling with a dying person obviously needs to be very gentle and appropriate to their needs. Enjoy it.

Moving a Person Who Needs Help

During a home dying, you'll have challenges helping the person move around, such as in and out of bed, to a chair, or to the bathroom or potty chair. Be sensitive to how much help the person needs. Over-helping undermines a person's sense of worth and dignity. Encourage the person to help him or herself unless it's too difficult or too discouraging. Move them the way they want to be moved. Support them in places they can't support themselves.

A visiting nurse can most easily demonstrate methods of moving a person, including a transfer belt. A transfer belt, usually made of canvas or nylon, is placed around the waist of a physically weak person to prevent their falling when you are helping them move, for example between bed and a wheelchair, or walking.

It's important to learn to move someone with the least amount of strain on yourself. One person can probably give all the support needed in the beginning. Later, you may need two. Here are some principles of healthy body mechanics when lifting and moving: whenever possible, keep your back straight; use thigh and stomach muscles; bend your knees and keep your weight over them; take a wide stance with one leg in front of the other with your weight evenly distributed; hold the person close to your middle, your center of gravity; don't lift a weight you can slide.

To help someone out of bed, imagine yourself in their place; sense what hurts and what's hardest for them about moving. Plan in advance with the person how you're going to lift or move them. What might get in your way? Any furniture or slippery rugs? Use non-skid slippers or bare feet.

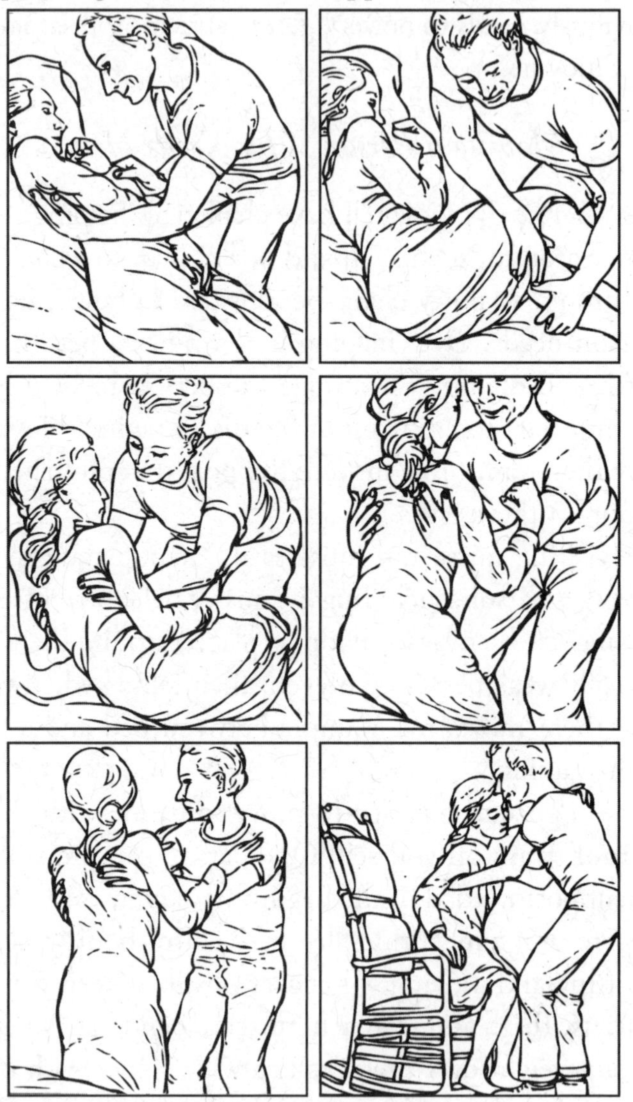

How to help a sick person from bed to chair. Awareness of balance and leverage is important.

If the person is moving to a chair or potty chair, place the chair at the side of the bed with its back facing the foot of the bed. When the person is ready to move, take a deep breath and relax. Relax your knees. If the move is to a wheelchair, make sure the brake is on and arm or foot rests aren't in the way. Then take the following steps:

1. Roll the person on her side, facing you. Drop the side rail if there is one.
2. If it's a hospital bed, raise the head of the bed.
3. Slide her legs partially over the side of the bed.
4. If she can't sit up alone, put one arm around the back of the shoulders, supporting the neck, and with the other arm gently pull her forward.
5. Stop a moment to let her get her balance sitting up. Make sure her feet are squarely in front of her.
6. If she can't help, face her, bend your knees, and put both arms around her, under her arms like a big hug. I sometimes put a hand under one buttock.
7. Brace one of your knees against her knee to prevent falling if her knees buckle, and gently lift her up (like waltzing).
8. Let her get her balance standing and, in this hugging "waltzing" position, move toward your destination.
9. If she doesn't need this much support, hold her under the armpits from the back.

To help a person in bed turn to their side: Raise the side rail (if any) and place one hand on the far shoulder and the other on the far hip. With your feet apart, gently roll the person toward you. Most patients can help by grasping the side rail or bed edge on the side they're turning toward.

To help a person move up in bed (toward the head of the bed): This can be done by one person if the patient is light or can help; otherwise, two are necessary. There are a number of possibilities:

1. If the person can help, have him bend his knees. Remove the pillows. Standing beside him, slide your arms under his back and thighs. Then, shift your weight forward toward the head of the bed as he pushes upward.
2. If the person can't help, use the same procedure as above, or two people can lift him with their arms under the head, shoulders, and hips.
3. A tug or draw sheet is a doubled sheet placed under someone from neck to buttocks. It's used by two people to move someone up or down the bed. Place it between the bottom sheet and the sheepskin pad, if there is one. Stand on opposite sides of the bed and roll the ends of the draw sheet toward the person in the center of the bed. Grip the rolled part firmly and lift-slide the person up or down. Be sure to support the person's neck.

After moving someone, help make him or her comfortable. Rearrange pillows and the pad between the knees and straighten the gown or nightshirt.

Remember "The Princess and the Pea"? People in bed are often super-sensitive to things we might not notice or feel. Some little irritation can make a person feel crazy if they can't move enough to do anything about it. As death approaches, you may have to move a person frequently. Trust your own loving tenderness. Relax and keep healthy body mechanics in mind so you don't strain your back. If you do (I have), don't be shy about asking someone for a massage.

Hospital Beds

A hospital bed has some advantages for the comfort of the dying person as well as for the helpers. You can easily elevate the person's head or knees to change positions. The height of the bed is adjustable so that the person's feet may touch the floor when they sit up, which makes getting in and out of bed easier. The adjustable height also helps prevent back strain for the helpers because they don't need to bend down as far to assist the person. Transfers from bed to wheelchair are also easier because you can make the two surfaces the same height. It's easy to hook up a trapeze to a hospital bed. A trapeze helps a bedridden person to lift the upper body or to turn himself.

The disadvantages of a hospital bed are it's not the person's own bed and cuddling is more difficult. Giving up their own bed is hard for many people. We used hospital beds with John and Mary. When Dad was asked if he wanted one, he didn't even bother to reply. He wasn't about to give up the bed he had shared with Mom for forty-three years.

If you reach a point when you feel a hospital bed would be less strain for you both, explain the advantages and ask delicately. Sometimes a little inconvenience is better than a change.

You can rent a hospital bed with electric or manual controls from a rental company. The manually operated ones are less expensive and perfectly adequate. On the other hand, being able to push a button when they want to change positions can help a bedridden person maintain some sense of control over their personal comfort.

Wheelchairs

A wheelchair gives a person who can't walk greater mobility and a change of scenery. Finding one is easy. Hospices, the

American Cancer Society, veteran's organizations, and other service groups loan wheelchairs, and rental companies rent them at reasonable monthly rates.

There are a variety of models, including one with a tray that locks in place if there's a concern your patient might get up and wander around. For me, having a very lightweight titanium wheelchair made my life much easier because almost daily I was loading it in and out of the car. If you have a choice, choose a model that most suits your and your loved one's needs.

To prevent accidents, make sure the brakes are on before helping someone move in or out of a wheelchair. See the illustrations for how to move a person from bed to wheelchair and back, or up and down a curb.

Memory Foam, Sheepskin Pads, and Pillows

Memory foam mattress toppers, sheepskin pads, and pillows are important aids for comfort and preventing bedsores.

Memory foam was first developed by NASA and then further developed for medical uses. Because it conforms to a person's body shape and weight-bearing areas, it reduces pressure points, thereby reducing pressure sores, or bedsores. A memory foam mattress topper is also very comfortable. Cover it with a mattress cover and a sheet. You can also purchase memory foam pillows and seat pads.

An artificial sheepskin is a washable synthetic pad about three feet by three feet. You place it under a patient from shoulder to buttocks. The pads are available from a hospital supplier and some fabric stores, or bring them home from the hospital. (You've paid for them!) Have several on hand: one for the bed or a chair, another to exchange for a soiled one.

Have extra soft, plump pillows available. For a change of

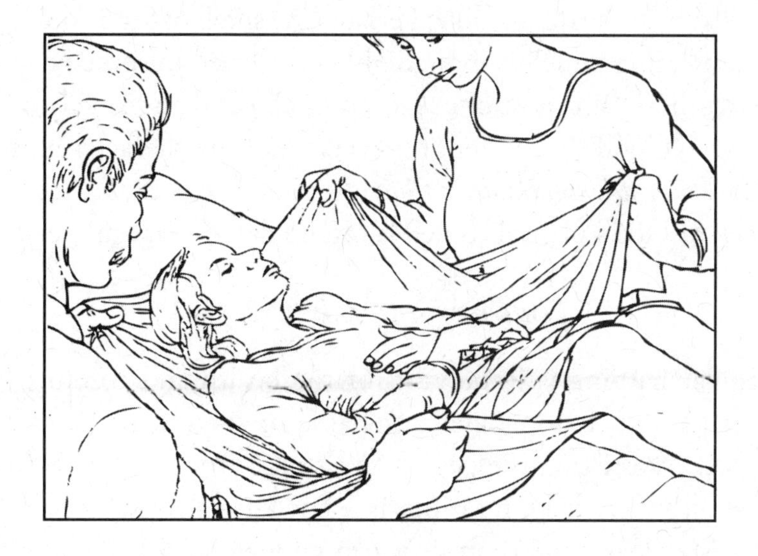

position for a person lying on her back, place a pillow under the knees to prop them up. For a patient on his side, place a pillow between the knees so they don't get raw from rubbing together. If a pillow feels too bulky, use a memory foam pad. Tucking a pillow in behind the back feels cozy and prevents rolling. Pile pillows at the foot of the bed under the top sheet to make a tent so the person's feet don't get tangled in the bedclothes.

You can also buy foam rubber wedges shaped like triangles. They're useful to position swollen ankles and calves to knee height, which alleviates some discomfort. Sheepskin or memory foam booties are useful to protect the heels of someone who's in bed much of the time.

SMELL

Cleanliness

What smells good when you're sick? Flowers, fresh air, sheets full of sunlight, incense, perfume? Ask your patient what smells she or he doesn't like. Perhaps the smell of food cooking is nauseating. Smell is more highly developed in some people than others, but most of us like to smell good and smell good things. "Good" is different for everyone! One character in the play *The Madwoman of Chaillot* loves garbage because "It's the smell of God's plenty!" Smell is often related to cleanliness.

Bathing and Changing

Regular bathing is important for the health and comfort of your patient. If someone can't bathe or shower, bathe them in bed. Is assisting the person to sit on a stool in the shower possible? Generally, morning is a good time for a bath, but ask. Make sure the room is warm enough so that chilling is not a problem. I use a natural sponge or cotton washcloth and a plastic pan for water. Find out what water temperature the person likes. Soaps without lots of perfumes and additives cause fewer dry skin problems. Have soft towels handy to cover the body parts you've already washed. Be sure to gently and thoroughly wash the genital area as odors collect there. There's no need to splash around so much water that towels are needed under the person, but place one next to the person to catch occasional drips.

After bathing, use a skin cream or lotion to prevent itchy skin. Alpha Keri is used by many hospitals, and there are natural products available at health food stores. Using baby powder around the genitals may prevent rashes.

After her bath, I gave Mary a short foot massage with cedar oil to stimulate circulation in her body. (Cedar oil is used by some Native Americans for purification.) If circulation is poor and the person has cold feet, put on socks or knitted slippers, or use a heating pad or hot water bottle. Remember to test the temperature and frequently check the areas touched by the heating pad or bottle.

Change gowns or pajamas at bath time and whenever necessary, yet not so often that it overly tires the patient. Gowns that open in the back are easier to take off and put on. Ones that go over the head are a pain in your back when the patient can't easily sit up.

Hair

For many of us, it's a treat to have someone comb and brush our hair, but for others, it's torture. Tangled hair can be uncomfortable, and who wants to look like a scarecrow? If visitors are coming, most people will want to look their best. It's also very satisfying to have clean hair. If a person cannot care for his or her own hair, you can do it. Brushing and combing may be part of a morning bathing ritual or done anytime.

There are several alternatives for cleaning hair. If patients can sit safely in a shower stall, you can wash their hair and bathe them at the same time. Hospitals generally use no-rinse shampoo: you pour a little on the hair, massage it in, and then towel-dry the hair. You can bring no-rinse shampoos home from the hospital or buy it at a hospital pharmacy. At a regular drug store, you can buy a shampoo that you spray on, let dry to a white powder, and then brush out.

You can also wash someone's hair in bed if you need to. Invent a system that works for you and the patient. Be well organized ahead of time because hair washing is very tiring for someone who is weak. You'll need a pan, towels, and plastic to keep the bedding dry.

If the person can't sit up, put pillows covered with a plastic trash bag and a towel under their neck. Check the water temperature. Then lean the head backward into a plastic pan to catch the water as you pour it through the hair. Gently towel-dry the hair. If the weather is cold, use a hairdryer to prevent chilling.

If you can't or don't want to wash someone's hair yourself, you might ask a beautician who's been trained to work with people in bed. You can locate one through a hospice, hospital, or visiting nurse association.

Note: Don't forget to cut the persons' fingernails so they don't scratch themselves. Some people enjoy a manicure, fingernail polish, or light makeup. A man may need help with shaving.

Teeth

Cleaning a person's mouth is important. It's awful to go through the day with "bottom of the bird cage" mouth. If toothpaste becomes too messy, you might change to hydrogen peroxide. If a person can't brush their own teeth, do it for them with peroxide on a toothbrush or Q-tips. Spongy swabs containing a special cleanser can be brought home from the hospital or bought from a hospital supply store or pharmacy.

Someone who wears dentures may want to continue using them. This is fine as long as they don't pose a danger. Consult a nurse or doctor.

Elimination

We need to bring all the compassion and caring we have to help people adjust to losing control of elimination. They usually feel ashamed and embarrassed. You might point out that the situation could just as easily be reversed; she or he could be helping you. Remind a mother or father of all the years they cleaned up their child. A cycle is completing itself, and we're reminded we're not just a body.

A catheter is one way to handle loss of bladder control. Another is placing a disposable cotton pad under the person, which also works for loss of bowel control. Disposable under-pads are available at medical supply stores and drug stores. Keep nightgowns or shirts out of the way and change the pads when necessary. Women can use a thick sanitary pad for extra absorbency. Men who dribble at night can lie on a shower cap filled with cotton balls.

After elimination, wash skin thoroughly and use powder or drying cream to prevent irritation or skin breakdown.

Not all dying people lose control of their bladders or bowels. If they do, they're generally on a bland diet with few animal products, so the smell isn't bad. If it makes you nauseous, put Tiger Balm or perfume under your nose and breathe through your mouth. Remember, this may be you later.

In the end, Mary and John were able to get to a toilet or potty chair. My dad used a bedpan once and lost control of his bowels once when he was drugged too heavily to wake up in the night.

As long as someone wants to and is able to get to the bathroom or potty chair (bedside commode), I suggest helping them, even if you think a bedpan or urinal might be easier for everyone. But do suggest a bedpan or urinal if getting to the bathroom or potty chair is so exhausting it doesn't leave much energy for more enjoyable activities.

People's feelings about maintaining their ability to take care of elimination can cause serious problems. At one point in our journey, I was Mom's only caregiver. She could walk very little, wore paper diapers, and at night there was a potty chair by her bed. I complained that I was getting exhausted getting up at night to put her on it and suggested she just wet her pants. Being a proud woman and being concerned about me, she got up on her own one night and tried to walk to the bathroom. She fell and broke her hip. Boy, was I sorry I'd complained!

Bedpans

There are two kinds of bedpans. The flatter kind (called a fracture pan) is easier to push under the buttocks. Bedpans along with plastic urinals for men are available from large pharmacies and medical supply companies.

To use one, roll the person to his side, position the bedpan under the buttocks, then roll him back onto the pan. Or, with a more mobile person, ask her to lie on her back, bend her knees, and bring her feet up as close to the buttocks as possible. Put one hand under the lower back and lift up as you place the bedpan under the buttocks with the other hand. Ask her to help, if possible, by pushing up the hips.

You might leave the room and ask to be called when they want to get off the pan. Flush the contents down the toilet and wash your hands.

Changing Sheets

Clean sheets are important to the well-being of the person you're caring for. A rubberized flannel under-sheet helps the mattress stay clean. Consider bringing outdoor freshness in by hanging sheets outside to dry in the sun.

Change the sheets whenever they're dirty, wet, sweaty, or if the person wants them changed. This may be several times a day or once every two or three days. You may save some changes by keeping towels around in case your patient spits up. Changing linens too often can be very tiring for you both.

If the person can't get out of bed, you'll have to change the sheets with them in bed. A visiting nurse can demonstrate how, or use these instructions:

Before any procedure directly involving your patient, explain what you plan to do and ask if it's okay. Have the clean linen handy before you begin.

1. Take off the top sheet and cover the person with a bathrobe or towel.

2. Roll the person onto his or her side with their back toward the center of the bed. Put the side rail up (on a hospital bed). Be careful the person doesn't slip off the edge.
3. Facing the backside of the patient, loosen the bottom sheet and roll it up until it's along his or her backside.
4. Position the clean bottom sheet on your side of the bed and tuck it in. Fold up the rest close to the rolled dirty sheet.
5. Help the person roll over both sheets to the side of the bed you've already fixed.
6. Move to the other side of the bed, pull away the dirty sheet, and tuck in the clean one.
7. Change the pillowcases.
8. Help the person back to the middle of the bed and put on the top sheet and covers.

Changing the sheets with a person in bed

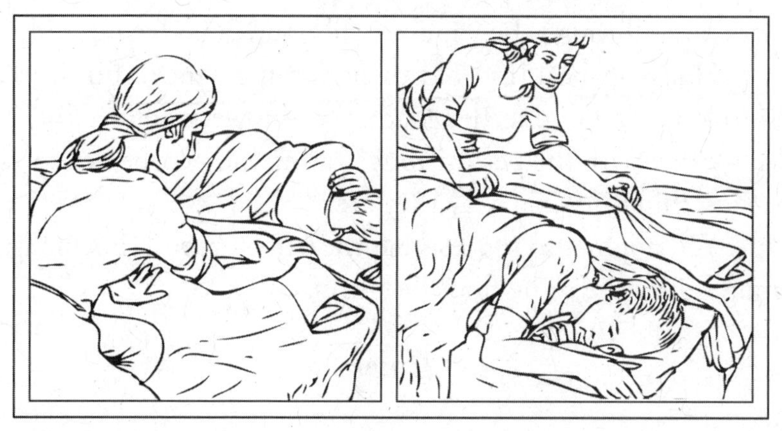

SIGHT

Beauty

Beauty heals. For a glimpse of the power of beauty, take a moment to remember how you've felt throughout your body when you've seen something you found incredibly beautiful.

Recent studies indicate that the pineal gland, whose function has not yet been scientifically determined, is stimulated by beauty.

In the past, the person you're caring for may not have made much time or space in his or her life for beauty. Perhaps you can help them open to an experience they may not have had before, so that in dying the adventure of life continues.

Imagine yourself in the place of the dying person. Try to experience his or her vision of beauty, and then do what you can to fill the room or home with it. Each vision will be different. To one person, beauty may be the old stained hat he always wore on fishing trips. Hang it up where he can see it. To another, it may be a painting, a weaving, or the way sunlight comes through an old lace curtain. If you have a choice, choose a room with windows so the dying can still experience the outside world: sky, trees, or the apartment next door. The sunlight that comes through the window will nourish body and soul.

Hang up beautiful old or new things, move furniture, add a lamp or a bird feeder. Gather wildflowers; go to a florist. Check first with the person you're caring for. Maybe beauty is leaving things just the way they are.

You might also suggest that the person spend time imagining things she or he finds beautiful.

Color

We're just beginning to remember the effect color has on us human beings. Play with color. Ask the person which ones she or he likes. Dying people often prefer the lightness of colors to the deepness—a rose or peach instead of deep wine. For me, for example, dying with a reddish-brown bedspread would be torture. Keep color in mind when you gather sheets, pajamas, nightgowns, bed-jackets, and bedspreads. If someone has a craving for a certain color, it means she or he needs it at some level of their being. To the extent you can, meet the desire for a color as you would a craving for a particular food.

Sunlight contains all colors, which is one of the reasons it nourishes us. If we're experiencing perfect harmony, we don't need more of one color than another. Most of us, though, need more harmony in our lives and could benefit from specific colors. This is particularly true for people with dis-ease.

There are many books about color and its relationship to different diseases and states of mind. Many don't agree on which color does what, so once again we have to trust ourselves and experiment. I recommend *Color Therapy*, by Reuben Amber. It includes the history of the use of color in healing, and practical ways to work with color.

Here are some general ideas to try. Greens through clear azure blues tend to be calming. Peachy pinks help depression. (Some say peach is the color of love of humanity.) The range of orchids, lavenders, and purples connect us to our spiritual nature. (Dad's favorite color when he was dying was purple.) Orchid relates to transcending matter. Some think cancer is related to deep grief, which is helped by greens, and lack of enthusiasm, which is helped by yellow, an emotional energizer. Orange vitalizes the body. If the dying person wants browns and grays, you might ask why. Those colors sometimes have to do with fear and pessimism, and your asking might bring up some unfinished business the person may want to talk about.

As you support this dying process, if you get a craving for a yellow dress or tie, treat yourself to it. There's usually enough money for what we really need, and "yellow" can be just as real a need as food or medicine.

Television

Lest I get carried away with beauty and color, TV is often a part of our visual lives. Ask the dying person if he or she wants a TV in the room, and if so, give them the remote control. If there's only one TV in the house, the person can still cooperate and sometimes watch someone else's favorite program. When someone's watching their favorite show, you might want to enjoy time alone.

Dad and I watched the world news together, and with Mary I used to insist on seeing *M.A.S.H.* because it made me laugh.

Here's another visual idea: Prominently display a photograph of your loved one when he or she was healthy. Perhaps the photograph can serve as a reminder to everyone that he or she, now gaunt and thin, is still the same human being and still deserves love and consideration.

HEARING

Sound

Sound has been used for soothing, purifying, and healing since the beginning of humankind.

"In the beginning was the Word, and the Word was with God, and the Word was God" (John 1:1). Does *word* mean "sound"? Many people are just beginning to be aware of sound's role in the creation. At some level we've all been aware of using sound to heal, such as lullabies, Native American chants in the sweat lodge, Gregorian chants in the monastery, and hymns in church. Sound and some kinds of music clear our minds so new energies can emerge.

At home the dying person is blessed with not hearing doctors' beepers and clanging meal trays. Enjoy the sound of silence. Enjoy the sounds of home: birds singing, a child laughing, the same old leaky faucet.

Experiment with giving the gift of sound to the person you're caring for. Would a bell help a weak person call you more easily? What about a CD player or iPod with some nature recordings of streams, whales singing, or ocean waves on a beach? Would hanging wind chimes outside the window be soothing? Some say chimes are the sound of the heart. They've been used for centuries in China and Japan. You can buy inexpensive ones at most import stores.

Music

What kind of music does the person like? Ask. It may be soul music, Bach, Beethoven's Ninth Symphony, or Mozart's "Ave verum corpus." What about flute music? Some say it's the sound of the soul. For many people, Pachelbel's "Canon in D major" is an old favorite. I like Georgia Kelly's harp music, *Seapeace,* and Steve Halpern's *Eventide.* You may know of, or discover, other healing pieces.

If you and the dying person have made music together, keep it up as long as you can.

Using the words appropriate for you, you might suggest that, as the person listens to music, he or she relax and breathe in the music, tune in to the harmonies. Music can be a needed break from the problems and routines of dying.

If someone seems to be holding in anger, it might be useful to play a piece of music you know she or he doesn't like.

It could help release the anger—and you'd have to be willing to take the consequences!

Reading to Someone

Reading is enjoyable for many people. Ask the person you're caring for if he or she would like to be read to. Reading can be a quiet, relaxing time for you both. When our attention is focused, not wandering among our everyday problems, other parts of ourselves are set free. Being read to also helps keep the mind active and prevents boredom, and it's not for everyone. Mary loved it. When I asked Dad if I could read him one of my favorite books, Allen Boones's *Kinship with All Life,* he didn't even answer, which was an answer.

What about storytelling, prayer, or meditation? Often there is time for just talking together about the things we really care about and wonder about.

Be sensitive to noises that may be irritating or painful to the dying person (e.g., banging doors, scraping furniture, vacuuming). Quiet is vital for healing and final preparation. Ask the person if there's too much noise or chatter.

Remember the sound of words of love. Use them generously.

TASTE

Taste is a sense some will enjoy right until the end of this life, even when other bodily functions have closed down.

From my present vantage point, if I were dying, I'd want Cadbury's chocolate instead of mashed carrots. This may change when my time comes! During Mary's last week she craved butterscotch sundaes (or her memories of them) and we ran out to get them. She could take only a few bites and generally spit them up, but she enjoyed the taste, so it was worth the effort. Dad craved raspberry sherbet and grape popsicles. Perhaps the digested sugar helped keep their minds clear.

Diet

Before terminal care, diet is very important. There are all kinds of different theories about purifying diets and about which diet is most appropriate for which disease. If you're interested, check a health food store for books. Do what the patient and you decide is best. You can always change your minds. If you give someone a certain food and later learn another could have been better, remember you did what seemed best at the time.

You may want to avoid artificial and chemically processed foods. When you're sick, your body has enough to deal with without the chemical preservatives and artificial coloring that the food industry uses. Fresh fruits, vegetables, and grains are usually appealing and easy to digest.

Once you've accepted that you're providing terminal care, consider giving the dying person whatever food he or she wants. Consider again the quality of life versus the quantity. It is possible that a reaction to a certain food might cause someone to leave a body earlier than expected.

If the sick person finds some foods unpleasant, it probably means he or she will have difficulty digesting them. If a person is indifferent to food, serve what's tolerable.

Chips of ice or iced drinks may reduce nausea and be refreshing. For a variety of flavors, freeze fruit juices in ice cube trays. If chewing is tiring, mash foods or put them through a blender.

If someone is on a liquid diet, make delicious, healthy combinations of fruit juices with yogurt, wheat germ, or powered vitamins. With a vegetable juicer, combine carrots, celery, and spinach. Straight carrot juice is wonderful—if the liver is functioning well. Create and experiment. Use a beautiful glass and straws that bend to make drinking easier.

Remember those grim hospital meals wrapped in cellophane on plastic trays? Even gourmet foods would look unappetizing presented that way. Serve food as attractively as possible. What about colored napkins, a drawing by a grandchild, a tiny racing car, or a flower on a food tray? For Mary, I used beautiful hand-painted plates with rabbits and cats on them. Beauty and music can soothe digestion.

Sick people often ask for a certain food and then can't eat it, perhaps because of nausea or blockage in the digestive tract. Remember that if you're caring for someone who can't eat, their difficulty does not reflect negatively on your ability to nourish. It just means that changes are taking place in the body.

For anyone accustomed to sharing love with food, watching someone she or he loves not eat can be very hard. For my mom, the hardest part of taking care of my dad was his inability to eat. The dying person can help by saying he feels loved even if he can't eat. Family members can help by suggesting other ways to share love, like massage or reading aloud, and pointing out that simply her presence radiates love. Dealing with your feelings when a loved one doesn't eat or eats very little is part of the process of letting go.

For in the dew of little things the heart finds its morning and is refreshed.

—Kahlil Gibran

10

LIVING FULLY WITH DYING: OUR FEELINGS

As we come more into the understanding that working with the dying is a way of working on ourselves, we find that working on ourselves means dying...letting go of the separate self, of every foothold and gesture that maintains our identity as apart from others and our original nature, our profound oneness with all that is.

—Stephen Levine
Author of *Who Dies?*

To live fully with dying we have to accept all of ourselves, including all our feelings—the ones we like as well as the ones we don't. Each feeling is a teacher.

Take time to *feel* your feelings. This may sound silly, but it's not. A lot of us ignore or run over our feelings in the rush to do the next thing. Then we're surprised when life feels meaningless or as if it's going too fast.

Supporting a home dying is an opportunity to slow down, to reappraise our values and to balance doing and being. When these elements are balanced, life regains meaning, mystery, and excitement. We then tap into a spring of limitless energy and have all the strength we need to support this dying person. Without the rest and nourishment of *being,* the constant activity of *doing* is exhausting. We make up for our backlog of fatigue by allowing ourselves to be. Then, to prevent feeling exhausted again, we can rest as we go along by being fully present for whatever we're doing or feeling.

Regaining this balance may shake up ideas and cause us to swing from one emotional peak to another. This is fine, a part of the process of surrender. We swing until we regain our balance—perhaps until we make a friend of death.

As you support this dying, accept the wisdom of your being; trust your feelings. After taking time to feel them, express them in a way that's appropriate for you. Once you've felt and expressed a feeling, you might want to experiment with sending love to the part of you that feels it: your angry self, sad self, impatient self, lonely self, disgusted self, or the child in you. Then let go of it. If you have trouble letting go, try taking some deep breaths or drink a glass of water. If you feel really scared or crazy, call a friend, counselor, or whomever feels appropriate. Do whatever you can think of to release the feeling, then breathe in peace. Make time to reflect on what your feeling may have been trying to help you understand.

Remember, the dying person is not the only one under stress.

The following feelings aren't in a particular order. If you feel drawn to one, go ahead and read it now.

HOPE

Hope is a reliance on the future that protects us from a "now" that is too painful. It's the question mark that is sometimes more desirable than an answer. As we walk through the darkness, hope may help sustain us.

It plays an important and complex role in the dying process. Nearly all dying people have hope in varying degrees, although the focus changes. At first they hope to regain their health, then to live a little longer, then to die an easy death. Hope is useful to sustain them through suffering, endless tests and treatments, being in bed, and losing control.

Don't crush hope in the person you're caring for. He or she needs it until acceptance is reached. Hope gives time to come to terms with impending loss. It can be both a sustainer and a form of denial. Whatever it is, we need to support hope and be truthful at the same time. For example, when first facing a terminal diagnosis, you might say, "Your tests don't look good but it's possible the treatment will reverse this" (if that's true). We can always encourage someone to hope to live well until he or she dies.

The idea that there may be a cure around the corner or a new breakthrough in treatments may help someone through a huge amount of discomfort. Breakthroughs are always possible. In the last couple of days before Dad died, he remembered with gratitude the doctor who gave him hope on the day, two years earlier, when he was first told he had cancer. The doctor said, "My mother's had cancer for the last ten years. It's not the end."

In her book, *On Death and Dying,* Dr. Kübler-Ross made two important observations about hope:

> *The conflicts we have seen in regard to hope arose from two main sources. The first and most painful one was the conveyance of hopelessness either on the part of the staff (hospital) or family when the patient still needed hope. The second source of anguish came from the family's inability to accept a patient's final stage; they desperately clung to hope when the patient himself was ready to die and sensed the family's inability to accept this fact.*[1]

When dying people express loss of hope, they generally die in a very short time.

LOVE

Our whole business in this life is to restore to health the eye of the heart whereby God may be seen.

—St. Augustine

Love is the worker of miracles that restores health to the eye of the heart.

Just now, if you wish, take a few minutes to slowly read the following meditation. It's even more enjoyable if there's someone else at home who can read it to you. Use this meditation any time you need some extra love.

> Remember some time in your life when you held and were held by someone you love: a child, a parent, a husband, a lover. Feel that again. Remember how soft and open and full you felt, how safe and comfortable! Remember what your breathing was like and breathe that way now. Feel the wholeness. Now give to yourself that love you were feeling. Give your love to yourself as you have given it to others; feel the fullness in your heart. There is a giver and a receiver in each of us that keeps the circle of love flowing. We can give and receive love inside of ourselves, as we give and receive love outside with others. Feel yourself surrounded and enveloped by love. It's there all the time, whether we feel it or not. Feel it giving you the strength you need for all the details, decisions, and maybe crises involved with this dying process you're supporting. If you feel heavy with worry, feel the heaviness lightening or lifting off. When we

> feel the love inside us, instead of looking outside for someone to love us, our own loving abundance makes everything easier.

As you support this dying, you will likely experience that love transcends and transforms time. One of the reasons we love to love is because it moves us beyond the ordinary limits of time. Recall the last time you felt a sense of timelessness. Perhaps you were with someone you love. The beauty and intensity of a relationship are often increased when we can see its end in time (death). Love, though, doesn't end with time; it belongs to eternity, and dying is leaving time for eternity.

The presence of love gives the dying person a supportive place and time in which to experience the incredible changes taking place within him or herself. When we bring someone home, we generally feel full of love; later, sometimes, it's difficult to maintain this feeling through tiredness, pressure, or complications. Sustaining love is easier if we are aware of who we are and where love comes from.

I'll share with you my reality or vision of who we are to give you a context for understanding what I say about love and fear. It's love and fear that are opposites, not love and hate. If there is truth for you in my reality, or any other, it will resonate in your own heart.

In the beginning was God (unity, energy), and God was without form. For God to have form, there had to be duality: a positive and negative charge. God created light and dark. The passive dark had no need to express, but the active light did. The part of God that wanted to express created humankind. The light is unconditional love; the dark is the space to receive it. When the light fills the darkness, there will be no more form. We return to God formless.

The formless Absolute is my Father, and God in form is my Mother.

—Kabir

Once we were created, we became attached to the form and forgot the formless. We forgot that God cannot express without us. Fear was created when the first human beings judged that duality and separation are the same thing. Fear, the illusion that we're separate from that which created and encompasses us, prevents us from remembering we are God and love in form.

When we remember, we experience no separation between God in form and God formless. We are both.

Life and death, to me, are a process of remembering we are an expression of God and love. Sharing in the dying of someone we love can accelerate our remembering. We've cheerfully acknowledged the devil in ourselves; maybe it's time to just as readily acknowledge the god in ourselves.

But if love underlies all of existence, why do I see cruelty, hate, greed, violence, guilt, and insensitivity all around me? Why do love and fear seem to go together? Why am I afraid to love? Why am I afraid to receive love? Why am I afraid when I do love someone—afraid I'll be hurt, afraid he'll leave me for another woman, be in an accident...or die? Why do I see unhappiness in my relationships and in those around me?

A possible answer is that, after we were created, we judged we were separate from love, felt afraid, and began to love conditionally. "I'll love you if you remember my birthday, if you dress the right way, if you have the right color skin, if you have the job I think you should have, if you'll never leave me, if..."

Unconditional love eliminates fear. Love is the absence of fear. Love is just, "I love you." "I love you, whoever you are, whatever you do, even if you leave me, even if you die. I love you without conditions and without expectations of anything."

Fear holds love a prisoner in the solar plexus, where it's a possessive feeling. When we dissolve fear by loving unconditionally, love moves up and opens the heart. When our hearts are open, we experience everything as love; there is nothing other. We've remembered who we are. We know love is the quality of our being, and we experience wholeness, or holiness.

When we love unconditionally, we take responsibility for our love. It's no longer dependent on another person—their presence, what they're doing, or what they might think about our love for them. When we take responsibility for our love, love connects us to joy, not to sadness and pain. And when someone we love is dying, we don't feel like we're losing our love.

We love by loving, not by talking about it or preaching. When we love the person we're caring for unconditionally ("I love you, even if you're denying that you are dying, even if you're afraid or angry or cranky"), we simultaneously love ourselves without condition. While loving others can open our hearts, to keep them open we have to love ourselves.

A common misunderstanding about love is that the heart is a container with a certain amount of love in it, and we can only give that amount. This is the idea of scarcity, that there's not enough love to go around. The heart isn't a container; it's more like a funnel that draws from limitless love. We can give more than we think we have and never run out. There's abundance, not scarcity. There's plenty of love for everyone.

Cruelty, greed, hate, violence, and guilt are fear's distortions of love, and so are healed by love. People like Mother Teresa, Martin Luther King Jr., and the Dalai Lama show us it is possible. My experience with dying people and women prisoners has taught me that unconditional love is the only thing that truly heals. When we love this way, we recognize who someone really is, beyond the limited set of beliefs and concepts they represent themselves to be. This heals.

One of the endless examples of the healing quality of love involved a young man with liver complications whom I visited only once. After fifty-six days in the hospital, no one could understand why he wouldn't let go and die. From his mother I gathered he hated himself because he'd been an alcoholic, had lost his job, and his wife and children had left him. I shared my beliefs with him: that I felt the purpose of a life-threatening disease is to help us remember who we are—love; that he was much more beautiful than his behavior, which was affected by a malfunctioning liver. I told him that at the deep level where all of us are one, I loved him. He died two hours later. The purpose of words is to love, to heal, and to serve. If you love somebody, tell them.

Once we remember we are love, we're responsible for living that truth in our daily lives by loving unconditionally. Don't feel badly or judge yourself if you don't do it all the time. We each love in the ways we're able to at each moment. We live with the paradox "everything is perfect" and "there's always room for improvement."

The great gift the dying give us is the opportunity to remember we are love, which is the same gift we can give to them.

COMPASSION

Unlike charity, which has taken on the connotation of doing something for someone to absolve a sense of guilt, compassion comes from putting ourselves in the other's place and knowing "There but by the grace of God go I." Unlike pity, which belittles both giver and receiver, compassion makes us both stronger.

When you're with someone who's dying, it helps you both if you imagine yourself in the dying person's place. The more we enter the world of the dying, the better we serve them and the more we learn. We're better able to understand a need for help with dry lips, a need to talk or to be alone, even a need that may seem ridiculous to us. We learn more about our own inevitable death, and although this may bring up our fears, in the long run it will ease our fear of dying.

Love and compassion will get you through unpleasant tasks like cleaning up if the person is throwing up or has lost control of their bowels. "I could be out of control like this and know that someone has to clean up after me." In the process of putting ourselves in the other's place, we're cleaning up our own life (and death) because we're not so likely to see ourselves as separate. And that could help change the world.

A student of Buddhism once asked his teacher, "Why does such terrible evil exist in the world?" The teacher replied, "Evil comes from ignorance. Evil comes from 'I,' from the mistaken idea that 'I' am separate from 'you.'"

Remember compassion for yourself. You deserve loving-kindness as much as the dying person does. We often remember compassion for others while forgetting we're due it as well. People often feel unworthy or think that's being selfish. It's not. We're more compassionate with others when we're compassionate with ourselves.

FAITH

What is faith? Unquestioning surrender to God's will.

—Swami Ramdas
Twentieth-century Indian philosopher and pilgrim

Faith is the belief of the heart in that knowledge which comes from the Unseen.

—Mohammad B. Khafif
Ninth-century Persian mystic and Sufi

For me, faith is trust in Life moment to moment. It's trust that whatever happens is part of an orderly harmony of all that is.

It's the knowing of the heart that transcends the thinking of the mind. The province of the mind is time; the province of the heart is eternity. To have faith, we need the larger vision. Religious beliefs may or may not play a part.

Faith allows us to feel peace and joy, even when we cannot understand what's happening in our lives. What appears to be separation, confusion, or chaos is transformed in the light of unity and perfection. We all have faith to some degree; otherwise, we'd stay awake at night worrying whether the sun will rise again. So it seems that faith alleviates fear and gives us more freedom to live fully.

Because faith is a knowing of the heart and we can't "know" in someone else's heart, it's useless to try to convince others to believe exactly as we do. Although we can share our experience, only their own experience can really convince them. Respect the faith of the dying even if it's unlike your own. Dying people quite often have visions or revelations that give them new or renewed faith that sustains them through the process of leaving the body.

A person who has little faith is not worse or better than one who has lots. All of us have different ways of learning. Doubt and cynicism are valid ways to learn discrimination. Discrimination may in the long run be the ability to look so deeply into things that we eventually see unity in everything.

Generally people who have chosen a rational/intellectual lens through which to see the world, or who think being in control is the most important factor in life, find surrender, giving up control, very frightening. At one time or another, and that may be at death, everyone learns surrender. Once we surrender and see that the sky hasn't fallen in, we may choose surrender again. Then surrender becomes an act of faith, not just hollering "uncle" because the pain is too great. Doubters and cynics gain faith from their own experience, not by accepting what someone else says they ought to believe. I call that integrity.

We have faith by choosing faith—and re-choosing it and re-choosing it. Each day, each moment, we have an opportunity to choose faith in unity or to choose to see separation.

Faith that dying is part of the breathing in and out of the universe, and not an end, facilitates the dying process. Dying is more easily accepted by a person who feels a sunset is not the end of the sun and shedding a body is not the end of life. Likewise, your work with a dying person is easier if you trust the rightness of the process. If you both have faith, dying can be a beautiful adventure into the little-known.

JOY

Joy is the essence of our being
The light that shines through us
The stars of our own recognition
It's the sun in our heart that reminds us
Life is as divine on earth as it is in heaven.
It's a candle that lights the darkness.
It's given us to remind us
Who we were before we were born.
The gift is always present.
It only waits for us to acknowledge its presence.

The joy I learned to experience while caring for John, Mary, Dad, Mom, and other dying people was unexpected. It was the joy that comes from being open to someone else and seeing yourself in them. A moment of spaciousness. A new awareness. An expansion of time. Nothing to do, nowhere to go, nobody to impress. Hearts opening. Two seemingly separate beings becoming one again.

I remember joy in seeing a shaft of light in a stairwell, being tucked in bed, loving someone and discovering they loved me, playing with seaweed, walking barefoot on dirt roads, and caring for my friends and parents when they were dying.

You may remember joy while playing in water bursting from a fire hydrant on a hot day, winning a race, painting a picture, celebrating the harvest, watching a shiny-eyed child running up the driveway, finding a solution to a tough problem, greeting a family member home from the war, childbirth itself.

When remembering joyful times in your life, recall how you felt: perhaps filled with a quiet radiance or as if a light suddenly lit up within you so bright that you could barely contain it. Joy is the spontaneous recognition of our wholeness or holiness.

Joy may be an unexpected quality of the dying process you're now living. It can be there if you allow it, if you do not make judgments that you shouldn't feel it.

If the person you're caring for is angry and looking for a target, you're likely to be one if you're radiating joy: "How can you be so happy when I'm here suffering?" We don't have to give up our joy for someone else. That's the old guilt con. You can explain that you're not happy they're suffering but that you are happy to be with them and caring for them. Nourishing your joy is part of taking care of yourself so you can live fully through a dying process.

Nurture your joy. Be a joyful servant. A very good way to say "good-bye" can be to live joy-fully.

GUILT

I told you I was sick.

—Epitaph on a tombstone

Guilt is a way we punish ourselves for learning, for not being perfect yet. It's a tool for manipulating ourselves and others.

Our culture's emphasis on both the past and the future promotes thinking like, "If I'd just done something differently in the past, things would be better now." There we go being the Monday morning quarterback of our own life!

The underlying pattern of guilt is, "To be a good person, I *should...*" We are intrinsically good, valuable, and worthy, and continue to be so, even if we never complete one *should.* The established *shoulds* may not be appropriate for our growth. If you complete a *should* that is not your own choice, you are giving up your power and choosing to be a martyr or victim. A martyr is someone who thinks suffering is noble, someone who doesn't act on what their body, mind, feelings, and soul tell them. They make themselves a victim.

Most of us divide our lives into two piles: what we *should* do and what we *want* to do. If we do what we *should,* we feel resentful and martyred or victimized. If we do what we *want,* we feel guilty. Perhaps a little voice says over our shoulder, "Irresponsible hedonist!" And so it goes. We bounce back and forth between the piles feeling split in two, and lead joyless lives.

To live joyfully and die contentedly or even just to grow, we have to stop splitting ourselves in two. The people I've observed who die the most contentedly, the most peacefully, are the ones who lived the most fully, who did more of what they *wanted,* without feeling guilty, and less of what they *should.* These wise teachers helped me understand, the only real preparation for death is to live life fully. Without regrets. Without I-wish-I-hads.

An alternative to dividing yourself in two and feeling partially alive is to do what you want to do, if it doesn't physically hurt others or their property, as long as you're willing to take responsibility for it. With freedom always comes responsibility. If you don't want to do something, and want to feel whole, don't do it or change your attitude. For example, you're caring for your dying wife at home. You want to get away, get out of the house, go to the movies. Go. Your feelings are the voice of your soul (consciousness) telling you what you need. They're not the tempting of some imaginary devil. When we cooperate with our feelings, the universe seems to provide the support we need. In this case, that might be someone to stay home with your wife or someone to drive you to the movies.

To continue the example, you get home from the movies, the supper dishes are still in the sink, and you don't feel like washing them. Don't. In the great scope of the universe, who really cares anyway? Certainly not the dishes. Or, perhaps you consider the bigger picture and think, "I need some outer order in my life now. I don't like the kitchen a mess or waking up to dirty dishes in the morning. I want to wash them now." You're then free to wash the dishes without resentment because it was your choice, not the choice of some invisible tyrant. Perhaps washing the dishes even becomes a source of quiet relaxation or a water game.

Again, a simple change in attitude changes our lives because our attitude determines the nature of our experience. The ultimate human freedom is freedom of choice of attitude.

"But, but, but..." I hear. "If everyone ran around doing what they wanted, life would be chaos." People want freedom, but they also want harmony and a certain amount of order in their lives. In my experience, doing what we want, as long as we take responsibility for it, doesn't create chaos. Life may feel a little chaotic initially as the people around us adjust to our getting stronger—to our ceasing to be victim to the terrible tyrant of *should* and reclaiming responsibility for our lives.

But in the long run, doing what we want creates not chaos, but increased harmony, strength, integrity, and respect for life. It encourages not irresponsibility but a deeper or wiser understanding of the meaning of responsibility. Responsibility, to me, includes acknowledging the sacredness of all of life. We're responsible not only for our outer life, but also for our inner life, including our feelings, and following their wise guidance.

Because guilt makes us feel separate from each other and God, self-forgiveness is one of the most important things we can learn. We need to be as loving and compassionate with ourselves as we are with others—perhaps more because we tend to be harder on ourselves than on others. Perhaps an important step in self-forgiveness could be to say "I forgive myself for anything I did that now seems unloving or unwise." Each of us is who we can be in each moment of our lives, and we can be open to change. Once we forgive ourselves, no one can flog us with guilt.

A dying situation often brings up feelings of guilt, although caring for someone at home helps prevent most of them. At home there's time and a place to express whatever you now feel or have felt in the past, thereby avoiding later regrets and remorse for not having said or done what you might have. If you have to take someone back to the hospital, nursing home, or hospice, know you are worthy even though a home dying is more than you can handle. "I should keep Grandma home" could be changed to "I'm a valuable person too, and I need help."

Besides not feeling guilty yourself, be careful not to make your patient feel guilty for dying. Saying "I could go to the store if I didn't have to wait to give you your medicine" or "Don't leave me with all this" makes a person feel guilty and/or ashamed. You should also be aware of a common pattern guilt takes: When we feel guilty about how we've treated someone, we often make them look bad in order to justify our treatment of them!

Being honest with the dying person helps prevent guilt. Honesty isn't ridding ourselves of guilt or getting ourselves off the hook at the expense of someone else. Guilt is also prevented by asking the patient what she or he wants whenever possible.

As I mentioned before, there's always the possibility you'll do or give something to the person that will result in their death before you expect it. If you've earlier agreed to do your best, and acknowledged you can't know everything, you may prevent useless guilt. Remember my giving the "liver flush" to Mary? Spare yourself a similar experience.

Be compassionate with yourself. Forgive yourself—over and over again. Instead of feeling guilt, congratulate yourself for outgrowing some old thought or feeling that is no longer appropriate for you, for increasing in wisdom.

Guilt, along with blame and punishment, are ideas we need to let go of if we want to live joyfully...or even survive.

HUMOR

There are no tortuous roads to climb, for an instant of humor transports a soul into another world, a bright hopeful world where anything is possible.

—A deva
Dorothy Maclean
To Hear the Angels Sing

A friend found W.C. Fields on his deathbed reading the Bible and asked him why he was reading it. Fields answered, "I'm looking for loopholes."

Humor can cause a smile, a tiny chuckle, or a big belly laugh. Enjoy it. It's a source of deep nourishment for your voyage. Humor gives perspective to a world where perspective is seriously needed. If we can laugh together, we may be able to cry together and more. We can become one again. Whenever possible, try to see the humor in the situation you're facing now. As long as humor comes from your heart, it can't be harmful. Only cynicism and sarcasm have a destructive side.

Remember Charlie Chaplin? Remember how he increased our compassion for one another and reminded us of our common humanity? We laughed because he lightly showed us our conflicts and our pomposity. Laughing can be a great equalizer; it opens the heart.

Humor usually helps unless we use it to escape our feelings. A joke is a new vision, not just a way to mask pain or discomfort.

Dying may be emotionally confusing for everyone involved. Humor helps us detach for a moment so we can see it more objectively. Humor helps the dying person deal with the frustration of needing help and not being able to do things she or he took for granted before. It helps make their situation seem less overwhelming and helps maintain a feeling of naturalness in the home. It releases blocked energies so we can see the larger picture. The details of life don't bog us down nearly so much if we laugh at ourselves, alone and together. We're really in a very leaky lifeboat, and we might as well enjoy it!

The belly laugh we had when Mary told us we were "rushing" her loosened the tension of many heavy days. The laugh we had when my sister told the priest that Dad was "somewhat Catholic" opened our hearts and released our fear. It would have been difficult to support them until they died without the lightening-up quality, the levity, of humor.

At a very deep level, humor heals.

Remember those funny family stories together, like the time Uncle John got caught...or Grandma found out...

Do you know why angels can fly? They take themselves lightly.

ANGER

A bull in a small pen is likely to kick the fence down.
A bull in a large meadow has room to move.

—Stephen Levine

Anger is an escape valve for the hurts and frustrations we pick up in the process of being human. We feel frustrated and hurt when we're attached to someone or something (life, for example) and things aren't going the way we think they should: "I'm angry because I hurt because Dad shouldn't die." Anger is a step on the way to surrender, a healthy sign as long as we don't hold on to it.

The amount of anger or rage or violence we feel is a measure of just how much hurt and frustration we're holding in. We can defuse anger by recognizing and expressing the hurt and frustration underneath it. We can transform it into compassion if we're willing to acknowledge we feel it. Many of us learned as children to hide our anger for fear of being punished for it. Now sometimes it's hard for us to recognize and/or acknowledge we feel it.

We transform anger into compassion by accepting that feeling angry is okay, by feeling and expressing the underlying hurt or frustration, and by accepting life as it is instead of holding on to how it should be. For example, the anger I first felt when Dad was dying was transformed to compassion only after I'd thrown some plates and rocks and cried and changed my thinking from "He shouldn't die" to "He is dying."

It's perfectly natural to feel anger when you're supporting the dying process of someone you love. Your sense of loss, abandonment, insecurity, feeling that this dying is taking too long, or feeling that the person should feel grateful can bring up anger. You may feel anger when someone says they want to live and you feel they're not really trying. What they may really be saying is not "I want to live" but "I'm afraid to die."

Sometimes with all this talk of acceptance and surrender, we feel angry if someone doesn't accept they're dying. Remember that people can die with dignity and be angry down to the wire. Perhaps that's a test for us. Do we really want them to die with dignity, their own way?

Let your anger out. The universe can absorb it. Our bodies can't. By not expressing anger, we hang on to control, and the price is high. We can't see very clearly from inside hurt or anger. Unexpressed anger can turn into nagging, irritability, depression, high blood pressure, and other serious illnesses or a big blowup later.

Freeing anger—accepting and expressing it—helps you and the dying person prepare for your loss and can help you both move toward acceptance. A dying person may not feel free to let go and die if people around are holding on to anger.

People often assume that expressing anger and hurting others are one and the same. It may be more hurtful not to express it. Protecting someone from anger says we don't trust them, that we know what's good for them. We're taking responsibility for their feelings and response, and assuming they're too dumb or unperceptive to recognize we're angry. In the long run, these things are a lot more hurtful than saying, "I'm angry with you. I love you and I'm angry."

If it's not appropriate for you to let out your anger in front of others, or you're afraid of the backlog of anger inside you, go off alone and bellow, throw balls, beat pillows, whatever you need to express yourself. If you have a wise friend or counselor, express the anger with them. Kübler-Ross suggested taking a foot and a half of rubber hose and beating on something you can't hurt until you can't beat anymore. For me, the side of the bathtub works. I prefer cleaning off black rubber marks to cutting myself off from joy later.

It's all right for people, even children, to see us angry. Children need to know anger exists, what it's about, that it's okay to feel it, and how to deal with it. You can explain to children that you aren't angry at them or the person who's dying, but angry because you're frustrated and hurt. Let them know you can love someone and be angry at the same time. Encourage them to let out their anger in a way that doesn't physically hurt themselves or others. Maybe you could go off somewhere together and throw rocks into a river, lake, or vacant lot. We lessen the amount of violence in the world by encouraging our children and everyone else to express their feelings.

I've heard people say about someone dying, "I'm angry because I love him so much." My response is, "Be angry. I know you love him. I know you hurt." Hurt was probably the immediate cause of the anger, and fear and loving conditionally the deeper causes (loving the person if she or he is here with me like I want).

We're moving toward loving unconditionally: "I love him, including his need to die."

FEAR

All know that the drops merge into the ocean
But few know that the ocean merges into the drops.

—Kabir

Dying and death may bring up more fear than any other circumstance of our lives. Supporting someone dying at home is an opportunity to face and accept this fear so we can transform it—and open wider our hearts.

Fear makes us feel alone, like separate drops that are not part of the ocean. It's caused by believing we are separate. Once we mistakenly believed we were alone and separate, we made judgments that confirmed our belief. Judgments are limiting beliefs that we have projected into the future and that prevent us from living without fear now. Our judgments prevent us from experiencing the underlying unity of everything that is.

For example, if your experience was "When I was seven, my aunt died, and I felt hurt and confused. Nobody would answer my questions, and Mommy and Daddy acted strange," the judgment probably was "Dying is terrible" or "I'm afraid of death." Even more likely, you didn't have a chance to experience that first mysterious death for yourself.

Parents' or friends' judgments—"Death is frightening" or "Dying is the worst thing that can happen"—were communicated verbally or nonverbally, leaving no possibility for you to experience dying and death for yourself. This is the way fear is passed from generation to generation. Your response to death from then on was probably controlled by a judgment you made at an early age. And all the judgments we've made in the past rule our lives until we consciously change them.

Descriptions, on the other hand, are not projected onto the future; they leave us free to experience the future as it comes. We can change a judgment—"I'm afraid of dying"—to a description. "Once my aunt died, and I was afraid. I don't know how I'll feel the next time." Or, "I know a lot of people are afraid of dying. I don't know how I feel because I haven't experienced it." Changing a judgment to a description leaves our energies free for the freshness of each new moment.

Fear creates what it fears. We attract everything that lies in our energy field. We attract what we fear in order to give us an opportunity to look at, understand, and release it. I was afraid of hospitals, blood, shots, sickness, and death, so I was drawn to work with dying people in hospitals, to transform those fears. Fear isn't "bad." It's just another teacher pointing the way home to more love.

If you feel afraid of dying or of anything else, don't override the feeling by insisting, "I shouldn't feel it." Our feelings and instincts help us select the experiences that are right for us; if we ignore them, we can end up with situations or people we don't like. Fear means we're not yet ready to accept an experience. Forcing an experience on yourself is not loving all of yourself. As long as you try to force yourself to accept something you're not ready to accept, you'll feel separate and will find it difficult to accept other people and their feelings as they are.

When you feel afraid, feel the fear and don't assume that's all of who you are. It may help to say, "Oh, there's that part of me that believes I'm separate, that *part* that is afraid of dying, of taking risks, of snakes" instead of "I am afraid of dying, taking risks, snakes." Send love to the part of you that feels separate and fearful and look for the judgment. Words like *good, bad, right, wrong, always, never, can't,* and *should* often indicate a judgment. When you understand the judgment, you can release it by forgiving yourself for making it, and change it to a description. The next time you run into the same old fear, experiment with focusing on love instead of the fear. Over a period of time, you'll find there are fewer things you're afraid of and you'll attract into your life fewer things you don't want.

We don't need fear. Fear is the absence of love. It can, however, show us where our love is needed. "But," someone says, "fear warns me of danger!" Isn't it awareness or instinct for survival, not fear, that warns us of possible danger? "But I have to teach my children to fear knives and cars for their own safety." Teaching with fear is one way. Another is to use love and patience to help children understand that knives are neither good nor bad. They're useful to cut sandwiches and, if used carelessly, they can cut us. We can help children understand potential dangers like knives and cars, and trust their survival instincts, or we can surround them with a miasma of our own fear. Using love and patience, we can help children understand dying without making it a fearful experience.

As you support a dying process, you may experience some of the fears of the dying person and some unique to being the one who remains behind in the everyday physical world. Your fear about what life will be like without this person you love, particularly in a husband and wife relationship, is usually matched by his or her concern for you. How will you mange the children or the business? Talking together about fears and planning possible solutions and alternatives eases the adjustment to life without the other person. Talking together may also help a dying person who feels afraid or guilty about deserting the family accept death.

Your fear of loneliness matches their fear of loneliness. While you're thinking, "I hurt because you're leaving me," he or she is probably thinking, "I hurt because I'm leaving you." Isolation, considered a major problem in the dying process, is greatly alleviated when you understand each other's fears and pain. Facing your fear or resentment now—"I'm not strong enough to stay here alone" or "I hate you for leaving me with this"—prevents remorse later.

Worry comes from fear about what's happening now or what may happen in the future. Worry goes on inside our heads. If you feel worry coming up, take a few deep breaths, relax, breathe love into your heart, see if you're doing the best you know, and let go of the rest. This will give space for a new idea or solution to come to you. Or it just may be that whatever you're worrying about needs to happen to give someone an opportunity to learn from it.

Remember, at each moment in our lives we choose, consciously or unconsciously, love or fear. And what we choose determines what we experience.

EMOTIONAL PAIN AND SUFFERING

Pain is the breaking of the shell that encloses your understanding.

—Kahlil Gibran

The amount of emotional pain and suffering around dying is directly related to the fear around it. Fear makes us resist what's happening or what may happen in our lives, and the resistance causes emotional pain. When we stop resisting, stop seeing the world as we think it should be, emotional pain lifts. Suffering is a habit of pain, sadness, or hurt. All of these are prevented and healed by accepting life as it is.

Pain is a useful message that something in our lives is not working. It's no longer needed when we pay attention to it, locate the resistance that caused it, and let go of it. When I was fighting against my dad's dying, I was in terrible pain. Holding on to him was obviously making me miserable. When I let go and accepted he was dying, I no longer hurt and was free to enjoy the time we had together.

Each journey to acceptance is unique; a lot of fear and arrogance made mine long and painful. Arrogance closes us to parts of life. Humility, being open to everything, makes the journey a lot easier.

While we're on our way, we need to be open to and accept our pain. Resisting pain just causes more pain; the pain is prolonged and becomes suffering.

If we grieve right away when we hurt, our pain is not stockpiled and doesn't become suffering.

If you're thinking, "Well, I don't want to hurt but I do," accept what you feel. You can't change the hurt until you acknowledge you feel it. So feel it. Express it in your own way. Love the *part* of you that hurts. Release the *should* that caused it. Some typical *shoulds* are "He shouldn't die," "She should love me," "They should do things my way," "Life should be happier," and "Pain, starvation, pollution, and war shouldn't exist."

If we accept our pain, we can accept someone else's pain. If we run away from our own, we'll run away from another's. Although we may be able to protect someone for a while, in the long run it's impossible to protect anyone from emotional pain. We need it and create it until we accept life as it is.

We often deny people the opportunity to learn surrender when we try to "jolly" them out of their pain. Have you ever felt like hollering at someone who was denying your pain? "There's no reason to feel bad," they say, or "You shouldn't feel so sad," "I know exactly how you feel," "By next week/month/year, you won't even remember." When someone says these things, people often respond with anger, which may distract them from feeling their pain and learning from it. Give the people you love a chance to feel their pain so they can learn from it and let go of it.

Taking on someone else's pain is as useless as denying it. Then two people, not just one, are suffering and the world is darker. Every time a heart is glad, it increases the light in the universe.

Taking on someone else's pain is one way to avoid feeling our own. It's something I did for most of my life. Only when we clean out our own reservoir of pain can we support someone in pain without losing energy and burning out. What, then, can you do for someone who's hurting emotionally? Have compassion and share love: "I know you hurt, and I love you." Once the person has felt the pain, if they're ready to release it, perhaps you can help them see what they're resisting and suggest alternatives.

There may be a part of ourselves that has an investment in our suffering: "If I suffer, I'm a good person." "I get a lot of attention when I suffer." "If I suffer, I don't have to take responsibility for my life." There may be a friend or relative who has an investment in our suffering: "If you were a good husband, you'd be suffering because your wife is dying."

We express love by loving, not by suffering. Suffering and emotional pain are not indispensable parts of the human experience. They're optional. No one forces us to resist the circumstances of our lives. God doesn't pin a medal on us because we suffer. Pain can help us to learn and grow, and it's possible to learn instead by awareness. If we pay attention, we may become aware of thoughts, people, or situations that might cause us pain before we hurt or when we feel a little edgy. Waiting until we're in agony before we pay attention is a hard way to learn!

It's possible to make a decision now, at this moment, in your heart to accept the circumstances of your life. Then you'd never have to feel emotional pain again (unless you started resisting again). This may not be probable, but for me, just knowing it's possible is comforting. As a friend of mine says about the idea of being free from pain, "That's scarier than infinity!"

Before John and Mary died at home, I thought dying was mostly about fear and suffering. There was much less of both than I expected. I found that sharing their dying, Dad's, and Mom's, and facing my own fear and pain opened my heart wider. I understand now that fear and pain have, all along, been a teacher about love and joy.

I know in my heart the day will come when we no longer need our old teachers. You and I, each in our own way and our own time, will graduate from the school of fear and pain and live joyfully on earth. I believe this dying you're sharing brings your graduation day closer.

I celebrate your journey.

All distinctions are false: The moment you say,
"This is good and that is bad," you have divided
life and killed it.

—Lao-Tse

11

LEGAL CONSIDERATIONS

An eye for an eye would make the whole world blind.

—Mahatma Ghandi

The legal considerations around a pending death reflect the degree of complication in a person's life. They relate principally to how a person wants to distribute the property she or he has collected. The laws governing property distribution are complicated and vary from state to state. I can most usefully familiarize you with some of the terms and procedures you may meet.

Help the dying person get their business affairs in order. If you're not asked, ask if he or she needs help. It's useful for the dying person to have a durable power of attorney (DPA), a legal document in which we name someone to do things for us if we can't. This authority might include the right to sign the person's name, and can be written to be general or for a specific purpose only. An ordinary power of attorney often becomes invalid if you become incompetent. A durable power of attorney remains effective, or in some states becomes effective, if you become incompetent. Because empowering others to make decisions for us is so important and state laws vary, you may want to ask a lawyer to advise and assist you in drawing up a durable power of attorney.

A joint bank account is also useful so you'll have cash available if you live in a state where bank accounts or other assets are frozen (can't be used) after a death. Locate, if they exist, the dying person's will, insurance policies, safety deposit box and keys, deeds to all properties and/or a burial plot, all securities, numbers of all bank accounts, automobile titles, pension plans, profit sharing plans, trust, copies of income tax returns, any power of attorney, individual retirement account (IRA), mortgage papers, and charge accounts.

ADVANCE DIRECTIVES, LIVING WILLS, AND HEALTH CARE PROXIES

Until recent years, most of us have counted on friends and family members to carry out our wishes about how we want to die. In our litigious culture, it has become obvious that we need to express our wishes in a legal form.

Advance directives are legal documents that protect our right to die in our own way. The two types of advance directives for health care are a living will and medical power of attorney, sometimes called a health care proxy.

A living will is a document we can sign in advance instructing that, in the event of a terminal condition, life-sustaining procedures be withheld or withdrawn. It gives us a voice if we can't speak for ourselves later. In the event of a legal, ethical, or medical question about treatment, it serves as clear evidence of our wishes. For insurance purposes, a living will is not construed as an intent to commit suicide.

A living will relieves both family and doctors of responsibility for making the ultimate decision about somebody else's life. By signing one, we perhaps give our loved ones a gift of peace of mind. Doctors feel safer about not being sued for malpractice.

In a living will, you need to clearly detail treatments you want and/or don't want if you are unable to express yourself, which is legally termed *incompetent.* Be specific. In the event of a serious or irreversible illness, do you want artificial feeding and fluids, antibiotics, chemotherapy, surgery, or cardiac resuscitation? Also, be specific about the condition or quality of life in which you would not want to be artificially maintained, such as permanent unconsciousness, severe dementia, or end-stage AIDS. If you want to donate organs and tissues after your death, include a statement about this in you declaration.

This legal statement must be witnessed by at least two adults unrelated to you and notarized to show the seriousness with which you regard it. Update the will every year by re-dating it and initialing the new date. Living wills can be revoked if you change your mind.

To additionally ensure that your wishes are followed in a terminal illness, it's useful to also complete a health care proxy, or medical power of attorney. In this document you name the family member, friend, or lawyer you want to make health care decisions for you if you are unable to make them. Also, you should name second and third choices in case your first choice is not available when you need him or her. In some states, a living will and a medical power of attorney may be one form; in others they may be two. In some states, a durable power of attorney serves the same function as a medical power of attorney.

Because advance directive forms vary by state, it's important to use the correct form. They are available from your doctor or local hospital, or you can download your state's form from the National Hospice and Palliative Care Organization at www.nhpco.org. You don't need a lawyer to complete these forms.

If the person you're caring for has not already made a living will or health care proxy, help him or her to do it. Once someone has signed advance directives, it's vital to inform family and friends. Be sure the people caring for the dying person know where it's located. Give a copy to his or her doctor and have one put in his or her hospital records. Give one to a clergy person if the dying person is close to one. One wise elderly woman, concerned about her wishes being followed regarding her end-of-life choices, taped her living will to her bathroom mirror.

In a home dying, sustaining life artificially is usually not a problem. It might become one if a person had to go into the hospital for a specific treatment and their condition worsened or they lapsed into a coma. Even if a person plans to die at home, making a living will can be useful.

If you are Catholic, you may already be aware that the June 1980 Declaration of Euthanasia concluded, "When inevitable death is imminent...it is permitted in conscience to take the decision to refuse forms of treatment that would only secure a precarious and burdensome prolongation of life." The United Methodist Church says, "We assert the right of every person to die in dignity...without efforts to prolong terminal illnesses merely because the technology is available to do so." The Central Conference of American Rabbis says, "The conclusion from the spirit of Jewish Law is that while you may not do anything to hasten death, you may, under special circumstances of suffering and helplessness, allow death to come."

See appendix B for a sample advance directive or below for a very personal creative one.

An Anonymous Alternative Living Will

"I, _______________, being of sound mind and body, do not wish to be kept alive indefinitely by artificial means.
Under no circumstances should my fate be put in the hands of pinhead politicians who couldn't pass ninth-grade biology if their lives depended on it. Nor in the hands of lawyers/doctors

who are interested simply in running up the bills.

If a reasonable amount of time passes and I fail to ask for at least one of the following:

Bloody Mary
Margarita
Scotch and soda
Martini
Glass of good wine
Vodka and tonic
Steak
Lobster or crab legs
The remote control
Bowl of ice cream
The sports page
Chocolate
Or sex

...it should be presumed that I won't ever get better.

When such a determination is reached, I hereby instruct my appointed person and attending physicians to pull the plug, reel in the tubes, and call it a day.

At this point, it is time to call a New Orleans Jazz Funeral Band to come do their thing at my funeral, and ask all of my friends to raise their glasses to toast the good times we have had.

SIGNATURE:____________________Date:__________

I also hear that in Ireland they have a nursing home with a pub. The patients are happier and they have a lot more visitors.

WILLS

A will is a legal document expressing how we want to distribute our material possessions and provide for our heirs upon our death. In legalese, a person who dies with a will dies testate, and one who dies without a will is intestate.

A will doesn't affect all the stuff you own. Property jointly owned, joint or "pay on death" bank accounts, insurance proceeds, Series E bonds, and death benefits like Social Security, VA, and union benefits bypass a will, but are counted for tax purposes.

Some of the advantages of making a will are choosing the person we want to administer distribution of our property (called the executor or personal representative), choosing who gets what (in case we doubt our survivors will follow our stated wishes), naming who will have custody of minor children, providing for an incapacitated adult, and lessening the possibility of future legal disputes over property ownership. A will can also be a love letter to our heirs.

A person with small children and no spouse will probably die more peacefully having made clear arrangements for their care. Instead of a blood relative, many people name as guardian the person most likely to love and guide the child to adulthood in a way consistent with the parent's views.

If the estate (what we leave behind) is small, a will is not always necessary, although generally advisable. If a person has a large estate, estate planning can save money in federal and state taxes. It's a complicated business that requires a knowledgeable lawyer who specializes in estate planning. To find a suitable one, ask friends or ask a trust officer of a bank, an accountant, or your local bar association to recommend one or more lawyers they consider qualified in this area.

A simple will takes a lawyer from one to four hours to prepare by the time she or he talks with you, drafts the will, and has it typed. An average fee for a simple will is $250. Before hiring a lawyer, ask how much he or she charges. Lawyers typically have consultation, hourly, and flat fees.

If after an initial consultation you decide to retain the

lawyer, reach a clear agreement on fees. If your income is low, check with a publicly supported legal clinic or your local bar association for no-cost or reduced-fee services. Online at legalzoom.com, you can prepare a simple will for less than one hundred dollars that meets the requirements of your state.

Valid Wills

What constitutes a valid will differs from state to state. For some of us it seems simple. It's a piece of paper Grandpa writes saying to whom he wants to leave what; however, the laws that determine the validity of a will place more importance on form than on content. A will must include property distribution, name an executor, and be signed and witnessed by two (sometimes three) people who sign in the presence of the author (testator) and each other.

A will may be partially or completely invalidated for many reasons:

1. The author was *incompetent* to make a will. (What legally constitutes incompetent varies by state.)
2. The author was *under undue influence* by other people. (Someone influenced the author to write the will in their favor.)
3. The will is not executed with the *formalities* required. (Each state requires formalities such as a certain number of witnesses, author must sign each page of the will, and witnesses attest they know it's a will they're signing.)

Most wills that are invalidated are invalidated because of the formalities. We have enormous latitude in the provisions of our wills, but not in the *form*.

Holographic Wills

A holographic will is one that is signed, dated, and written entirely by hand by the author. It must include disposal of property and in some states must name an executor. Some states require a witness while others don't. A holographic will is recognized as valid in the following states: Alaska, Arizona, Arkansas, California, Colorado, Idaho, Kentucky, Louisiana, Maine, Michigan, Mississippi, Nebraska, Nevada, New Jersey, New York, North Carolina, North Dakota, Oklahoma, Pennsylvania, South Dakota, Tennessee, Texas, Utah, Virginia, West Virginia, and Wyoming. Maryland will recognize a holographic will as valid only if it is written by a member of the armed forces.

This type of will is usually written in an emergency situation. But, if you live in one of these states and don't own property in another, you can write your own will, although a lawyer would not recommend that you do so. A person who has property in more than one state needs a lawyer. In some of the states listed, it may be possible to type or dictate a holographic will. Check with the court in your area that has probate jurisdiction.

No Will

A lot of people die intestate, without a will. When people die without a will, their property is distributed according to the law of intestate succession or the law of descent and distribution of the state in which they live. Property jointly owned, life insurance proceeds, and death benefits bypass the law of intestate succession.

Under laws of intestate succession, property generally goes first to the surviving husband or wife, then to their children, and then to other blood relatives. If you care who gets your possessions, it's a good idea to find out the law in your state so you don't create problems for your survivors. A legal clinic or lawyer can help you.

In some states, for example, if you have a wife and one minor child, the law distributes half of the estate to your wife and half to the child. If the child is a minor, the court will name a guardian, who is normally the surviving parent. But the guardian may have to put up a bond (post money) and *must* get permission from the court to spend any of the child's money, and must file an accounting with the court each year. This means time, money, and nuisance for the guardian that can be avoided by writing a will, perhaps with trust provisions. A *trust* is an agreement between you and a financial institution or person to handle money or property for you.

For the enjoyment of it and/or to avoid dealing with lawyers and courts, some people simply give away their property before they die. Legally we must file a federal gift tax return on all gifts given to one person worth over $11,000 per year (or $22,000 per year if the spouse agrees). Each year we can give tax-free gifts of this size to as many people as we choose. If one gives larger gifts and dies before filing the tax return, the executor is responsible for filing it.

The Executor or Personal Representative

The executor or personal representative is the person named by the writer of the will to take charge of his or her financial affairs and distribute property after death. If there's no will, an administrator-executor is named by the court. The work of the executor may take up to a year or two if the estate is large or complicated. She or he is paid by the will writer's estate for the work done. The payment varies by state; it's a "reasonable fee" or a percentage (1 to 5 percent) of the estate.

The following discussion of the legal responsibilities of the executor is excerpted from *Law for the Layman* by attorney George G. Coughlin:

1. *He (she) may take the assets of the estate into his (her) possession. (This means the executor takes control of the assets of the estate and obtains full information about all the deceased's belongings. She opens a bank account in the name of the estate and transfers the deceased's account to her name as executor. She collects the proceeds from insurance policies if they're payable to the estate (otherwise the money goes directly to the beneficiaries) and looks after stocks and bonds. Executors need to keep detailed records of all financial proceedings.)*
2. *He (she) may sell and liquidate personal property and convert the assets of the estate into cash. (If cash is needed to pay debts, the executor can sell personal property and real estate.)*
3. *He (she) may pay debts and funeral and administration expenses. (This involves placing a notice in newspaper that any creditors of the deceased present their claims. If state and federal taxes are due, the executor is responsible for paying them.)*
4. *He (she) may distribute the estate to the beneficiaries. (After all debts, expenses and taxes have been paid.)*

PROBATE

Probate is the name used by the courts for the administration of an estate, which includes opening and closing it. It documents legal ownership of inherited property. According to Phillip Stern, author of *Lawyers on Trial,* "Probate is up to 100 times more expensive here than in England, and that's because England has 'de-lawyered' the process. In this country we end up paying two and a half to three times as much in fees to probate attorneys as we do in funeral expenses."

Probate is necessary if a person dies with a will or without a will if the property includes such items as real estate, stocks and bonds, or bank accounts that must be passed on according to the laws of intestate succession. Probate is not necessary if a person leaves no will and only owns property of the sort that bypasses the law of intestate succession, like earlier-mentioned jointly owned property, joint or "pay on death" bank accounts, insurance proceeds, Series E Bonds, and death benefits like Social Security, VA, and union benefits. Also, accounts with beneficiaries such as insurance policies and 401(k)s go directly to the person named. Legally, personal effects and clothing may be subject to probate, but in practice they're generally divided among family and friends.

When someone dies who has a will, the person named in it as executor, or a lawyer versed in probate, takes it and a copy of the death certificate to the local court with probate jurisdiction and files for probate. The judge then decides if the will is valid. If someone dies without a will and there is property that doesn't bypass probate, then the closest relative, friend, or their lawyer takes the death certificate to the court and files to be named administrator. The judge decides the proper person for the job. Whoever is appointed may be required to post a bond to guarantee they'll do a good job and won't run off with the loot.

Once you file, the court issues letters testamentary if there's a will, or letters of administration if not. The letters state that the executor accepts responsibility for collecting assets, paying debts and taxes, distributing the property, and closing the estate.

The executor lists the assets collected, the debts, inheritance taxes, and the share of each beneficiary. If there are no disputes, the property is distributed to the beneficiaries; they acknowledge receiving their share and the estate is closed. If there are disputes, the estate can be settled by written agreement among the disputing parties, or the executor and the people involved go before the judge for a decision. Upon proof of distribution, the estate can be closed.

TAXES

Depending on the size of the estate, state and/or federal taxes may have to be paid. Taxes vary from state to state. A few impose none.

A federal tax return must be filed on any gross estate that exceeds a certain amount. *Gross estate* means everything someone owned, or retained some control over, and even includes some property such as insurance that bypasses probate. The tax return must be filed and is due within nine months of the death, although you can apply for an extension.

According to the political winds, the amount of an estate exempted from federal tax varies greatly ($600,000 in 1987 and $3,500,000 in 2007). In 2010, the estate tax is completely repealed, and in 2011 the estate tax law returns to using 2001 rules, except that the exemption goes to $1 million. No one says this has to make sense![1] The federal estate tax exemptions change, so check the amounts with the IRS, a tax preparer, accountant, or tax lawyer.

If the estate in question is of any size, consult an attorney or accountant about estate planning. Estate planning is about seeing that a person's property is well managed, properly distributed, and saves money on taxes. Tax accountants, bank trust officers, and estate-planning lawyers are the people to consult if the finances involved warrant it. They know, for example, how to use trusts, marital deductions, and similar devices to "split" an estate so that upon the death of the husband or wife, federal estate tax will be lowered or the estate will be exempt from taxation. Many of us who aren't knowledgeable about taxes think owning everything in common when we're married is the loving way to handle property. However, for people with a large estate, joint ownership may be unwise because it increases the estate taxes that may be due in the future.

BODY DONATIONS

In recent years, all states have enacted or revised Anatomical Gift Laws, which permit people to donate all or parts of their bodies to hospitals, research, or educational institutions.

If you or the dying person want to give your body or parts of it, tell your family, write a letter stating your wishes, and fill out a Uniform Donor Card. Call a medical school or hospital to get exact details for your state and area. Ask if your age and physical condition are suitable. The presence of cancer or a communicable disease disqualifies a transplant donor, except for corneas.

In many states, Uniform Donor Cards are on the back of drivers' licenses. I recommend consulting with The Living Bank, a national nonprofit organization. They will not only supply you with a card, but also the address and phone number of the federally funded organ procurement organization for your state. 1-800-528-2971 or e-mail info@livingbank.org.

Uniform donor card:

UNIFORM DONOR CARD

of ______________________________

(Print or type name of donor)

In the hope that I may help others, I hereby make this anatomical gift, if medically acceptable, to take effect upon my death. The words and marks below indicate my desires.
I give:
(a) __ any needed organs or parts,
(b) __ only the following organs or parts

____

(specify the organs or parts)

for the purpose of transplantation, therapy, medical research, or education
Limitations or special wishes, if any:

____

UNIFORM DONOR CARD

Signed by the donor and the following two witnesses in the presence of each other:

____
Signature of Donor — Date of Birth

____
City and State — Date Signed

____
Witness — Witness

This is a legal document under the Uniform Anatomical Gift Act or similar laws. For futher information, contact the New England Organ Bank 1 800 446-NEOB or the Center for Donation and Transplant 1 800 803-6667

This card is recognized in all states and musts be signed by two witnesses.

Nothing is more or less sacred than anything else.
Everything and everyone are equally divine.
—From a meditation

12

HEALING

At the core of healing is a deep mystery that is to be respected. It is the mystery of transformation and regeneration and is different for each person. It is the mystery of balance and harmony, and at the core of this mystery lies the universal Heart.

—Satya Miriam
Healing Is Transformation

I share with you my beliefs about the nature of our being, of disease, and of healing. Throughout the world, increasing numbers of people are coming to the same or similar realizations. They're departures from a lot of old assumptions.

Each of us is a whole composed of body, mind, feelings, and soul. Body, mind, and feelings are sometimes called the "body," or the personality of the soul. The word *personality* comes from the Latin *persona,* which means "mask." The soul is consciousness, spirit, or God, individualized. Disease (dis-ease) indicates a disharmony within the whole. The body is the last part of us in which dis-ease manifests. It appears first as a disharmony between the soul and mind or feelings. To heal, we have to understand and treat ourselves as whole beings within a physical and social environment.

At present, most medical, or allopathic, doctors are trained to treat the symptoms of disease rather than to support an individual's own process of healing. Penicillin and aspirin, for example, are not going to heal a person's real dis-ease. At best, they buy time by curing symptoms so we can discover and heal the real imbalance. Splints may help cure a leg broken in a car accident, but they won't heal the consciousness that caused the person to be in the accident. Curing symptoms and healing dis-ease aren't the same thing.

The more we've given away the responsibility for our health to doctors, the sicker we've become. It's not the doctors' fault. We're the ones who got addicted to the body as our main point of reference and mistakenly look for the source of healing outside of ourselves. The source of healing is within. The work of medical doctors can be very valuable but has limits because it works only on physical symptoms, or, in the care of psychiatrists, with mental and emotional symptoms. Real healing must take place at *all* levels of our being.

Healing, or righting the energy balance within us, is a process that requires our active participation. Human beings are dense, somewhat solidified energy. An imbalance in this energy results in disharmony or disease. It can be a great adventure to find the source of the imbalance and to heal ourselves. The dying person you are supporting can certainly be healed—even if his or her body cannot be cured or saved. Sometimes the fundamental imbalance is healed and the body dies anyway.

Many people have lost faith in prayers (an important healing aid) because they prayed for someone to be healed and she or he died. I believe our prayers are heard. Perhaps we don't recognize the answer. The disharmony in the person may be healed and yet it's time for him or her to leave a now uninhabitable body. Prayer is useful if we avoid praying for what we want and pray instead for whatever is the highest good for ourselves and others. We're fortunate if we know the divine plan for ourselves, let alone for someone else.

We are either victims of our diseases or we are responsible for them. I believe we're responsible. This is much more hopeful and useful than thinking we're victims. If we're victims, disease is out of our control and we can't do anything about it except try to cure the symptoms. On the other hand, if we're responsible (accept our dis-ease as ours), it is possible to help ourselves.

The principal pitfall when we begin to take responsibility for our disease is guilt. Who needs to feel sick and guilty too? For many years my body was sick with one thing or another. For four of those years after I was introduced to holistic healing and began to take responsibility for my sickness, I felt like a spiritual leper. I didn't want to see anyone because I was sure they'd see I was sick and know something was wrong with me spiritually. I felt sick and guilty—and I was afraid to talk with anyone about it.

Spare yourself! There's nothing to feel guilty about. The body is a sacred vehicle and messenger. If the postman brought you a letter that contained information you didn't want to hear, you wouldn't berate the postman or feel guilty. When our bodies give us a message that something is not working, instead of berating ourselves, we can thank our bodies, send them love, take care of them in the ways appropriate for us, and start looking for the source of the imbalance.

Within each of us is soul and personality, masculine and feminine, giver and receiver, pragmatist and visionary, do-er and be-er, father and mother, creator and inspiration, light and darkness, intellect and intuition, movement and rest, will and awareness. When we balance these polarities, we feel vibrant, alive, and whole. If we neglect any of them, we cause an imbalance in the whole—dis-ease. We can balance them by accepting, nourishing, and expressing them. The marriage of the polarities within us is the most important marriage we make. It opens our hearts and connects us to our source.

To find the source of the imbalance, we must find the part or parts of ourselves that we do not love unconditionally. When body, mind, feelings, and soul are not in balance, we limit the amount of God (or energy) we can express, and we're not aware of who we really are. If we accept only body, mind, and feelings, we accept only half of ourselves, of God. If we accept only soul, we accept only half. When we accept both, we're truly healthy and whole.

You may want to look at the polarities in your own being. Are you listening to both your visionary and your pragmatist? Are you using your intellect as well as your intuition? If you're a man, are you expressing the feminine qualities in you? If you're a woman, are you expressing the masculine qualities in you? Are you allowing time for quiet and time for activity, time for creating and time for inspiration? Are you as good at receiving as you are at giving, and vice versa? Are you loving and accepting all of yourself?

When you make the two one and when you make the inner as the outer, and the outer as the inner, and the above as the below, and when you make the male and the female into a single one, so that the male will not be male and the female not be female, then shall you enter the Kingdom.[1]

—Jesus Christ
The Gospel According to Thomas

We can recognize imbalance when we see sickness instead of health, fear instead of love, hate instead of compassion, separation instead of unity, war instead of peace. Imbalance exists when we don't see matter and spirit as equally sacred, and when we don't accept life as it is. Balance comes from changing what we can and leaving the rest to be transformed in its own time. An imbalance exists if we don't remember "Not my will, but Thine."

What can you do if you find you have a life-threatening disease? The following suggestions are adapted from an anonymous contributor to *New Age Magazine.*

1. Avoid medical paraphernalia and practices that treat only symptoms—unless, of course, you need to buy time to heal the source of the disease. (Chemotherapy and radiation don't heal cancer. In large amounts they destroy the immune system, which must be strengthened in order to heal ourselves.)
2. Sit down and center yourself. Begin reversing the self-irresponsibility pattern endorsed by the culture and ask yourself, "How did I create this situation? Do I really want out? Of life? Of the disease?" If it's life you want out of, acknowledge that cancer, for example, was the one-way ticket you purchased and it's okay. If you decide you want out of the disease, then accept that any condition you have created can be recreated. Any decision you have made can be reversed.
3. Take a holistic approach. A superior healer, to use the Chinese phrase, uses modalities that support the healing forces of the patient; the inferior healer uses modalities that fight disease. Locate a superior healer.
4. Use your experience as a learning and growth vehicle by extracting the principles involved. It's not enough to live. Survival as a life purpose is mockery. The body, like a fine musical instrument that must be kept in tune in order to be useful, might occasionally need repairing and turning. When it no longer responds to repairing and tuning, it should be discarded as graciously and as soon as possible. Clutter diminishes the clarity of living.

You may want to consider healing possibilities you haven't tried before or you may want to stay with the familiar. Whether you prefer holistic or traditional medicine, get a second opinion and consider alternatives. There are unskilled practitioners and charlatans in both groups. To discriminate which treatment forms are appropriate for you, research the alternatives, use your intuition and intellect, and choose from the heart.

Barry Sultanoff, MD, psychiatrist, offers these wise prescriptions for all of us "suffering" with dis-ease.

1. *Breathe. Quiet yourself, observe your breath, count your breaths. Reflect on the marvelous process of breathing.*
2. *Ask for help and express your willingness to receive it. Ask a friend for a backrub. Ask God, your higher self, for healing on whatever level serves your highest good.*
3. *Forgive others and forgive yourself.*
4. *Listen to healing music.*
5. *Sing, hum, chant, yodel.*
6. *Laugh. Ask people to tell you jokes and funny stories.*
7. *Ask your "inner child" what to do about your symptoms and what she or he needs from you. Take time to play.*
8. *Write or telephone someone you feel "at odds with." Express your willingness to let go of positions or attitudes you held about them in the past. Ask what he or she wants from you.*

9. *Take a walk in nature. Observe and ask yourself, "What does nature have to teach me about how I can heal myself?" Ask trees, flowers, birds, or animals you meet along the way, "What can you tell me about...?"*
10. *Hug as many people as possible, as often as possible. Say "I love you" to yourself and to others.*

The following list includes additional tools that can be used to create a healing path unique to each person.

Allopathy	Homeopathy	Music therapy
Yoga	Do-in	Dancing
Herbs	Shiatsu	Drawing
Rolfing	Polarity therapy	Dreams
Feldenkrais	Psychic surgery	Rebirthing
Vitamins	Chiropractic care	Bach flower remedies
Diet	Aikido	Meditation
Jogging	Biofeedback	Affirmations
Acupuncture	Gestalt therapy	Astrology
Massage	Encounter	Tarot
Color work	EMDR	Guided meditation
Sound	Aura balancing	Prayer
Art therapy	Tai Chi	Spiritual healers

I've often observed people begin to experiment with alternative techniques and become discouraged when they didn't get the desired results. Either the person didn't work on all levels (body, mind, feelings, and soul) or didn't know that a person can be healed and no longer needs a body. Healing as an intellectual pursuit alone doesn't work.

Two useful survey books on natural and holistic healing are *Prescription for Nutritional Healing,* by Phyllis Balch and James F. Balch, MD, and *The Practical Encyclopedia of Natural Healing* by Mark Bricklin.

ENERGY WORK

Until you have experienced working with energy, it sounds a little like hocus-pocus. Once you've experienced it, it becomes real, like other things we can't see: electricity, laser light, and radiation. Perhaps learning about energy work is another case of needing to suspend judgment in order to learn something new. In my experience, it's a very effective healing technique.

Light is one name for the energy that created and sustains us. Some physicists believe that we, and everything else, are made up of tiny strings of light. To metaphysicians, *Light* is another name for unconditional love, the life force, the Christ, Buddha, Allah, etc. When we call in the light (become conscious of it), we become a container and channel for it as long as we remain focused on it. And the purpose of calling Light in is to support healing.

If you want to support yourself or another, you might ask the Light to be present. I ask that "The Christ Spirit" be present. Use whatever words suit you. There's no need to tell this energy what to do because it has perfect knowledge. Ask that it be used for the highest good of whomever you're sending it to, so you don't interfere with his or her process or your own. You may feel it or see it as a light coming through the top of your head and filling your body. No effort is needed. When we exert ourselves, we have no place to receive. At first you may feel a little dizzy and uneasy. This passes as your body adjusts to the energy. You may feel nothing special at all, but that doesn't mean it's not working.

"Holding the Light" means remaining focused in your heart, for whatever amount of time feels good. This may be a few minutes or a half hour. At the same time as you hold the Light for another, you are also being healed. I find holding the Light very supportive for dying people and continue to do it periodically during the first weeks after death.

Reiki and Healing Touch are other forms of energy work. Many hospital nurses have been trained in Healing Touch and find it helps their patients to feel peaceful and relaxed.

LAWS FOR HEALING

Three universal laws for healing are "As above, so below," self-forgiveness, and "As we think in our hearts, so we are."

"As above, so below." If perfection exists in the universe, it exists in us as well. If there is love, beauty, health, peace, and joy "above," or anywhere else, they are in us as well. Lifting the blinders that prevent us from seeing them is simple and not easy.

The blinders are our judgments, our limited thinking: "This is good (or bad)"; "This is right (or wrong)." Everything is energy, and energy is neither right nor wrong. It just *is.* There is only one energy from which everything is created. It can be used skillfully or unskillfully, with love or with fear. We make judgments that make things seem separate, and then we feel separate. A human being, table, flower, and bomb are all manifestations of the one energy. We have free will to use energy as we choose.

Self-forgiveness. God, or whatever you like to call this underlying energy, doesn't judge and so has nothing to forgive us for. We judge ourselves, so we must forgive ourselves. We need to forgive ourselves whenever we make judgments that make us feel separate or less than who we are. Perhaps that's many times a day. Each time we forgive ourselves, our hearts open wider. "I forgive myself for being afraid I don't know enough to write this book." "I forgive myself for thinking there's not enough money for my needs." "I forgive myself for not loving myself and others more." "I forgive myself for fearing fear."

Self-forgiveness is an art we learn as we move toward loving ourselves and remembering who we are. If you need help with forgiving, I recommend *Forgiveness, the Greatest Healer of All* by Jerald Jampolsky, MD.

"As we think in our hearts, so we are." If we think we're sick, we're sick. And we're free to change our thinking. If we think from our hearts, we're healthy. If we think from our hearts, we know love, joy, peace, beauty, and abundance. Even if we just focus on these qualities with our minds, we make room for them to develop in our lives.

Each day we can choose what we think and whether to think from our divisive minds or from our unlimited hearts. When I find myself running around my mind in negative circles, I use a technique called EMDR, which stands for the mental mouthful "eye movement desensitization and reprocessing." It's a short-term therapy that helps heal anything from negative thinking to post-traumatic stress disorder. If you are interested, you can explore EMDR online.

If your body is sick, you might ask your friends to think of and visualize you as healthy, not sick. A lot of friends thinking of us as sick can hold us to old patterns and help us stay sick.

A person with cancer can visualize each cell working perfectly and any malfunctioning cells lifting up and out of the body. Again, remember to work at the feeling, body, and soul levels as well. Carl Simonton, MD, has worked extensively and successfully with nutrition and visualization techniques for cancer. Excellent instruction tapes as well as an award-winning video, *Affirmations for Getting Well Again,* can be ordered from his web site.

A GUIDED MEDITATION

Guided meditation is another way to explore our inner experience and capacity for healing. Earlier, I mentioned that a transcendent or mystical experience can eliminate or transform pain. Guided meditation is a simple method of helping someone get in touch with their own transformative energies, whether or not they're in pain.

I have used the mediation below with many people. If this meditation isn't appropriate for the person you're caring for, you can create your own. You may give or receive a guided meditation. Don't be upset if the person cries. People often do. Some people fall asleep, and that's all right also. Both times I used this meditation with Mom and Dad, they fell asleep about the time they got to the "top of the mountain," and they woke up feeling great!

Ask the person to lie down or sit, making him- or herself as comfortable as possible. Keep your voice soft and non-interfering. Leave time—long pauses—as you read for the person to get images and experience his or her feelings. The meditation is as follows:

> *Close your eyes and breathe gently. With each breath, gently move deeper inside yourself. Imagine that you're in a beautiful meadow. The sun is coming down in golden rays through you and around you. (If the person is in pain, suggest, "As you feel the sun, allow its light to move through any place in your body that hurts, any place in your feelings that hurt. Start relaxing the tension around the hurt. Imagine each cell around the*

area softening, opening, relaxing. Keep softening and opening and letting the light fill you." Then continue.)

Open fully to the light and let it fill you. Relax and feel the richness around you and through you. Smell the air. Touch the earth and feel it in your hands. Are there birds or flowers or animals? Be with them. You feel perfectly comfortable with everything. Is there a stream or brook? If so, listen to the sound of the water. Are there any wild berries, wild strawberries, or anything to eat? If so, put it in your mouth and really savor it. If there is anything you want to do in this meadow where there are no limits, do it: explore, sing, dance.

On the other side of the meadow is a beautiful mountain. Start walking toward it and climbing up it. If you need help, imagine something to help you: a bird, a person, an elevator. You can imagine anything you want. You can see that the light at the top of the mountain is incredibly beautiful. As you climb, light starts to fill you. Soon you're at the top. If you need a rest, invent a seat. An exquisite beam of light surrounds you and fills you; allow yourself to really feel the light. Within the light, a figure or form comes toward you that represents the highest you know. You feel this being's love for you; really let that love in. (Allow plenty of time.) You know that this person or energy has always loved you and has never judged you or anything you've done. Forgive yourself for all the times you've judged yourself or other people, for all the times you've felt unworthy, guilty, fearful.

As you forgive yourself, feel your heart opening wider. Forgive yourself for all the judgments you've made against your body, your feelings, your mind. Allow forgiveness and love to fill every cell of your being. If you like, ask the figure or energy any question you have about anything. The figure or energy reaches out to you and gives you a gift to take with you so you can remember this experience. After you receive the gift, say good-bye, knowing you can always return.

From the top of the mountain, take the light that fills you and radiate it to everyone: all the people you love; all the people, plants, animals; all the creatures of the earth. When you feel ready, slowly come down the mountain with your heart open, bringing this light energy with you. Take all the time you need; there's no hurry. When you feel ready, open your eyes, bringing the energy back into this room.

Allow yourself to receive and share whatever the person brings back.

Butterflies count not in months but in moments and have time enough.

—Rabindranath Tagore

13

PREPARATIONS FOR DEATH AND AFTERWARD

For brief as water falling will be death.

—Conrad Aiken

SIGNS OF IMMINENT DEATH

As the moment of death approaches, a dying person usually wants more and more time alone, resting and sleeping, preparing internally for what is to come. Cells are dying at a greater rate than ever, and the person has less and less physical energy. As you see the person less connected to the outer world, it is better if there are fewer visitors and external distractions.

You may find it nourishing at times to just sit quietly and watch the dying person. Silence is a living, healing energy that makes space for renewal and internal preparations. One friend said, "I know why I was sitting with my father. It was so my heart could open wider and I could feel his essence." Your intuition will tell you if gentle touching is a comfort to the person or an intrusion.

Don't misinterpret a dying person's seeming distance or lack of connectedness with you as a lack of love. Even as he or she loves you dearly, he or she is beginning to move toward the new life. Share this with family members whose feelings might be hurt. While death is easy, dying can be hard work.

Dying people are often conscious until death. Some move into a coma. Although medically they're called unconscious, they're not. As I said before, a person in this state hears everything at some level. Talk in their presence as you would with a conscious person, not as if they were unconscious. We are alive and have consciousness even when very little or nothing is functioning outwardly.

If you have unfinished things to share with someone in a coma, talk to them and know they'll hear you. Questions may be fruitless because the person can't answer verbally. Although, if you listen with your heart, you may hear the answer. One way to understand a coma is as a kindly teaching that we're not just a body.

The dying person will take less and less food and liquid. Less urine will be eliminated. If she or he can no longer eat or drink, keep the mouth as moist and fresh as possible. Remember, use ice chips or a wet washcloth to suck on.

If the person is dehydrated or the air is very dry, mist the room with a spray bottle filled with water; any empty spray bottle will do. Some people enjoy having their bodies sprayed with a water mist. Ask. Personally, I like using rose water spray.

One sign of approaching death, but not necessarily imminent death, may be an odor coming from the person. To me, it seems to be the smell of cells decaying. If there are lung complications, the odor may be particularly strong. With cancer, a strong odor is sometimes present earlier. In John's case, the odor was so strong that some of us felt nauseated. Burning incense and putting Tiger Balm under our noses helped. BENGAY or a light perfume works as well. A different odor about my mom was what initiated Li'l Deb calling me right before Mom died. In my father's case, by contrast, there was no odor.

A person in the last stages of dying may find massage soothing, or an intrusion or interruption. Use your intuition. A very gentle massage may be one of the last outward ways of expressing our love. Dying people are sensitive to pressure. A person with cancer may be quite "skeletal" by now, with very little fleshy protection for the bones. (Remember, pillows and padding between the knees.) Because the skin is also sensitive, use a cream skin toughener if you have one. I've used Lanacaine and oil prepared by a herbologist containing benzoin and myrrh. Sensitivity to light may be heightened. If you need a bright light to see by, warn the person so they're prepared for it.

As people approach death, their arms and legs may get colder and colder as circulation withdraws. Keep them warmly covered. Some people sweat profusely. If they do, lighten the covers. Don't tuck in the top sheet or covers, so the person can move about if able to. Put some pillows or folded blankets at the foot of the bed, under the sheets, to make a space for the feet to move easily. Again, you may be asked to turn the person frequently, which can be exhausting and may take two people. Most people close to death need less pain medication.

Other possible signs that death could be near: the underside of the body becomes a darker color, the mouth hangs open, brown secretions in the mouth (possibly old blood from the stomach lining), the pupils of the eyes react less to changes in light. The person may have a glazed, faraway look or stare into the distance without blinking. In sleep, the eyes may shut only partially. If you take a pulse, you may notice it's weak. The skin may be pale and waxy and the face drawn. Again, even if the person is showing few signs of life, talk in their presence as if they're present, because they are.

As a result of changes in body metabolism, the dying may experience increasing confusion about time, place, and identity of family and friends. Reassure them by telling them the time, a person's name, or who's in the room. Loosening connections here is part of the preparation for death. It's important not to insist that they pay attention to what's "real" for us, which may no longer be for them.

It's not uncommon for dying people to talk out loud with God or someone who's already died. Dad saw lights around him. Many people report seeing relatives and friends who died earlier. Some people call this "hallucinating." The word suggests they're crazy or need sedation; they aren't and they don't. I believe they've just opened the door to another level of reality. On this level they may have a profound mystical or religious experience. The dying may also experience various degrees of age regression and relive important memories or review their entire lives. Respect these preparations. If their words seem garbled, listen carefully. You may discover unsuspected meanings that may help you meet a final need and/or comfort you.

As a person moves close to death, breathing usually becomes more and more labored. Secretions may build up in the lungs so that less oxygen is being exchanged for carbon dioxide, further weakening the person physically. You can help them by speaking gently and soothingly, or just by breathing gently and fully yourself. You might ask the person to remember how they breathed sitting or sleeping next to someone they love and suggest they breathe that way now.

Even closer to death, the breathing pattern may change again. A drastic change in breathing doesn't necessarily mean the person is going to die immediately. A person may continue for a number of days to breathe in a way which might suggest each breath is the last. The breathing may seem bizarre and frightening if you're not used to hearing it. There may be a crescendo of breath and then no breathing for ten to thirty seconds. Doctors call this Cheyne-Stokes or neurogenic respiration.

You may hear a rasping or gurgling sound at the back of the throat caused by oral secretions that the person can't cough up. For the sake of the family, hospices often use a Transderm Scōp, a medicated Band-Aid placed behind the person's ear that eliminates the sound by drying up the secretions. You need a doctor's prescription for it. Elevating the person's head may help ease the effort of breathing.

If the breathing bothers you, take breaks out of the room. The breathing may not only sound strange, but also bother us because we feel helpless. Perhaps the deeper reason for our discomfort is that by now we're seeing the difference between the person we love and his or her body. When we see the body hanging on, we may feel a sense of inappropriateness. Could you be watching the labor pains of the soul?

The symptoms of imminent death given here may not all appear at the same time and some not at all.

Dying people know at some level when they're going to die. Both Mary and Dad communicated that they knew, and Mom sure knew how long she had to hang on before getting to the doctor's office to die. Using your intuition is one way to know when death will come. When John was dying, I meditated and prayed for guidance and was told he had four days. On the fourth day, he died. Don't worry if you're off. Life's timetable is flexible.

Whether or not a person has accepted that they're dying, there is frequently a period of peace before death; perhaps it's the final surrender. It's interesting to note that according to Ruth Gray, a nurse and author of *Dealing with Death and Dying,* "A dying person always turns his head toward the light."

Could it be that as we die we know we're going home to the Light even before we open the garden gate?

BEING WITH SOMEONE THE LAST FEW DAYS

A dying man needs to die, as a sleepy man needs to sleep.

—Stewart Alsop

During the last few days, it's most useful if your attitude is one of letting go and releasing the person. Both of you are working on surrender, trusting the moment. Suffering is caused if a person is ready to die and feels the family is hanging on. It creates a struggle. "I know I can't stay, and I don't feel like I can leave." Let the person know you'll be okay and encourage him or her to go free.

Two situations that may come up at the end of a dying process can generate a lot of guilt if we misunderstand them. The first is a feeling of irritation or anger that this process is taking too long. It's a natural feeling many experience, like a mother who loves her child yet is tired because she or he needs so much attention. Recognize the anger or irritation and forgive yourself. These feelings are signals that we need a rest, a change of scenery, time away for ourselves. The person is still here because he or she has something to finish on some level. It'll be easier for you if you don't make assumptions about how long the process will take and continue to pace yourself.

The second situation occurs if the death happens while you're out of the house or room. If someone wants to feel badly because "I wasn't there," that's a choice. Not being present may also be a beautiful expression of love. Many dying people are so attached to people they love that it's easier for them to die when those people are not present. The energy of loved ones can hold us in a body we need to leave.

Perhaps you have to leave town before the actual death. We are no less loving or loved because of our physical location. We can tell the person before leaving that we love them and know they love us. And an appropriate expression of our love is to live the life we are given to live. Even if this never reaches words, we know that love is not expressed only by sitting at the bedside.

A PRACTICE MEDITATION FOR LEAVING THE BODY

When we sense that death is near, all we can be is present. Quiet. Loving. Open. Holding hands if that feels appropriate. Suggest she or he breathe as calmly as possible. I suggest (verbally or nonverbally) that the person move toward the Light, allowing him or herself to feel lighter and lighter, lifting up.

Perhaps the meditation, or parts of it, that follows may be useful for you before the actual time of death. At the moment of death, silence may be more appropriate. Read the meditation to yourself first. If it feels appropriate to you, ask if the dying person wants to try it. For some people, it's clearly inappropriate.

It's not probable that a person will leave their body during the meditation, but it's possible. If the body dies, it's because it's time. Remember, the vehicle does not die until after the soul decides to withdraw its energy. This meditation may be used as is, or you may be inspired to create one based on your own beliefs.

(The person's name), we love you and we're ready to let you go. Feel a lighter body within your heavy physical body; move into your Light body. You don't need the old one anymore. Trust each moment. Let go of any distractions or anything that's holding you here. Softly and lightly. We're okay. Surrender to who you are. Feel our love, God's love. We are love. If there is anything you haven't forgiven yourself for, forgive yourself now. (pause) You may review your life so that the lessons are clear. There is no punishment, only unconditional love.

We are One and we can never be separated. Move into the Light. Just keep moving into the clear Light. Nothing to cling to...

Whenever it feels right, just lift up and dissolve into the Light. There's no pain, only Light. Anything you see is a projection of your mind. Think God. See Light. "Be not afraid, for I am with you even in the shadow of death." Move from the shadow into the Light. You will see and hear us. Don't be surprised if we can't hear you when it's your time to leave. The veil will not yet have lifted for us. You'll be met and welcomed on the other side, and God will comfort us.

You're going Home. Home is the brightest Light. Move into the brightest Light. Know we love you and rejoice for your homecoming. You are free, home to the one heart, total understanding, beauty, joy. We are One.

THE MOMENT OF DEATH

We use the phrase "moment of death" because that's how long death lasts: just a moment.

Signs of death may be no breathing or heartbeat, loss of bowel and bladder control, no response to shaking or shouting, eyelids slightly open, eyes fixed, and/or jaw relaxed and mouth slightly open.

The sound of silence may be the most loving gift right before the moment of death. At this moment, people of the Jewish faith say, "Baruch Dayan Ha-emet" (Blessed is the Judge of Truth); others say "Glory to God," or chant "Om." At the moment of death, the final thread holding the life force to the body releases. There is no pain. Consciousness leaves the dead body. I've experienced the life force lifting up out of the body through the solar plexus, the heart, or the crown of the head. If you place your hand over these places at the moment of death, you may feel the energy going out. Your hand will tingle or feel different.

IMMEDIATELY AFTER DEATH

Do whatever is right for you and your faith tradition.
Be who you are. Be your heart. Share your hearts.
Pray, perhaps for God to help _____ to his or her new life.
Close your eyes and see what you see. Close your ears and hear what you hear.
Allow your tears, your grieving.
Breathe deeply, exhale deeply.
Hold someone who needs holding. Be held.
Send your blessing with the newly free.
Send love to all around you.
Chant or sing a prayer.
Does anyone need extra help?
Make a circle holding hands and linking hearts.
A silence of thoughts.

LAYING OUT THE BODY

Treat the body with respect, knowing, however, that it's only a body. What you do with it in terms of cleaning and dressing has to do with your needs, not those of the soul now free. Dressing the body is easier in the first hours before it starts to stiffen. Unless you want to, it's not necessary to dress a body for cremation, for going to a hospital for an autopsy, or to a funeral home. We dressed Mary and John ourselves and didn't find it gruesome—just another task to be completed with love. Dad had promised the doctors at the VA hospital that they could examine his body so we didn't dress it. I've observed a hospice volunteer or nurse dress a body for the family.

In choosing clothes, think of what the person enjoyed wearing and how they'd like to be last seen. If a man was not a coat-and-tie type, it adds a jarring note to see him decked out like a Wall Street businessman or like an attendant at someone else's funeral. It doesn't matter what some relatives or friends may think. They can do it their way when it's their turn.

If it bothers you to see the eyes open, close them shortly after death. If the aesthetics of an open mouth bothers you, tie the jaw closed with a scarf that goes under the chin and ties on top of the head.

After death, the body may involuntarily empty its bladder or bowels. Remember, it's a function of the body that is no longer related to the person. It doesn't always happen.

A short time after death, the faces of John, Mary, and Dad looked more relaxed, peaceful, and younger than while they were dying. All signs of the effort of leaving had gone.

There's no need to spend a lot of time with a body. Yet I recommend spending enough time so you really know it's only a cocoon. Go into the room where the body lies as often as it feels right. Perhaps talk with the person; encourage him or her to go free.

When you feel ready, call the funeral home, if you're using one, to remove the body.

GETTING A DEATH CERTIFICATE

To prevent legal complications, you'll need a death certificate signed by a physician, medical examiner, or coroner. If a doctor is present at the death and has the certificate, he or she can sign it right away.

If a doctor is not present, call the one you've been working with. If you don't have one, call the medical examiner or coroner.

A doctor usually has to see the body before signing a death certificate. If it's the middle of the night, wait until morning.

If you're working with a hospice, they'll help you get the death certificate. A hospice nurse can pronounce someone dead. If the nurse is present, she or he will call the coroner's office and report an expected death at home. The coroner gives the time, which is stated on the death certificate. The hospice nurse calls the funeral home, and the funeral home picks up the body. The funeral home sends a death certificate to the doctor and returns it to you.

You will need copies of the death certificate for the state, banks, insurance companies, etc. Keep the original.

ADVISING RELATIVES AND FRIENDS

Advising relatives and friends of the death and burial plans should be done promptly in case they need time to get there. It's helpful to have a list of phone numbers and addresses ready. You might want to do the actual calling or be grateful for a volunteer. However, if no one has had any sleep, all this can wait until the next day. Sleep.

A CHECKLIST OF THINGS TO DO

The checklist shared here is adapted from *Dealing Creatively with Death: A Manual of Death Education and Simple Burial* by Ernest Morgan. Some of these things need to be done shortly after death and others may be done by you or friends and relatives in the weeks to come. Not all will apply to you.

_____ Decide on time and place of funeral or memorial services.

_____ Notify immediate family, close friends, and your employer or business colleagues.

_____ Arrange for family members or close friends to take turns answering the door or phone, keeping a careful record of calls.

_____ Arrange appropriate child care.

_____ Coordinate the supplying of food for the next few days.

_____ If flowers are to be omitted, decide on appropriate memorial or charity to which gifts may be made.

_____ Write the obituary. Include age, place of birth, occupation, college degrees, memberships held, military service, outstanding work, list of survivors in immediate family, or any other information you want to share. Give the time and place of memorial services. Deliver to newspaper by telephone or e-mail.

_____ Notify insurance companies, including automobile insurance, for immediate cancellation and refund of premiums.

_____ Consider special needs of the household, such as cleaning, etc., which might be done by friends.

_____ Arrange hospitality for visiting relatives and friends.

_____ Select pallbearers and notify them. (Avoid ones with heart or back difficulties, or make them honorary pallbearers.)

_____ Notify the lawyer and personal representative (executor).

_____ Plan for disposition of flowers after funeral. (Leave them on the grave or give them to a hospital or nursing home?)

_____ Prepare a list of people living at a distance to be notified by letter or printed notice, and decide which to send to each.

_____ Prepare the message or printed notice if one is wanted.

_____ Prepare a list of people to be acknowledged for flowers, calls, etc. Send appropriate acknowledgments. (May be written notes, printed acknowledgements, or some of each.)

_____ Check carefully all life and casualty insurance policies and death benefits, including Social Security, credit union, trade union, fraternal, military, etc. Check also on income for survivors from these sources.

_____ Check promptly on all debts, mortgages, and installment payments. Some may carry life insurance clauses that will cancel the debt. If there is to be a delay in meeting payments, consult with creditors and ask for more time before the payments are due.

_____ If the deceased was living alone, notify utilities and landlord and tell the post office where to send mail. Take precautions against thieves.

Bury me if you can catch me.

—Socrates

14

PLANNING A BURIAL AND SERVICE

The goal is to allow the body at death to rejoin the elements
it sprang from,
to use what remains of a life to rejuvenate new life,
to return dust to dust.

—Mark Harris
Grave Matters

A simple analogy for death Kübler-Ross often used is a butterfly leaving the cocoon. In a burial and memorial service, consider focusing on the beauty of the living butterfly instead of on the cocoon.

If possible, make burial plans ahead of time. It may be more difficult to make practical decisions after the death than before. If you're feeling less than calm, you're more likely to let others—like the funeral industry, friends, clergy—take responsibility for arrangements. If you can't plan ahead, don't worry. You may be surprised how everything falls naturally into place.

Find out your state's law about how a body can be disposed of. Call the county coroner, state board of medical examiners, or a local memorial society. (See the section below, "To Dispose of a Cocoon"). In John's and Mary's cases, all we knew ahead of time was that our state law permitted burial on private property.

When Dad was dying, we talked with him and without him about plans, and my mother visited several funeral homes.

I called the San Antonio city coroner to find out the Texas laws. Embalming was not legally required, so we planned to have his body refrigerated, the coffin closed, and no visitors to the funeral home.

My parents' home was in a little incorporated city within San Antonio, so I also called the local courthouse. The police chief said they had to investigate any death at home, but because they knew Dad and what we planned, it wouldn't be necessary. A simple call avoided a police visit.

Police are required by law to investigate a "medically unattended death." In many places, they also investigate a natural home death attended by a doctor. Having police come into your home right after the death of someone you love is emotionally jarring, so preventing it, if possible, is worth a try. Again, find out the legal requirements in your area.

In some places, a police visit after such a death is a tradition, not a legal requirement. In those places, you might avoid one by calling, ahead of the death, the police and/or medical examiner (coroner). Let them know what you're doing—preparing for a natural, expected death at home attended by a doctor—and ask their advice about preventing a police visit. You might ask your doctor, hospice, or funeral home director to make the call for you. If a natural, expected death at home is not under the jurisdiction of the police or medical examiner, simply don't call them or emergency medical services (EMS) after the death. If a police visit is unavoidable, ask the person most able to handle such a visit to answer the questions the police are required to ask.

Let's look at the purpose of a burial service to enable you to create a meaningful one that nourishes you and fulfills the purpose.

1. To dispose of a cocoon.

2. To facilitate the process of grieving by allowing family and friends to express their love for the living spirit of the dead and for one another.

TO DISPOSE OF A COCOON

Only when the earth shall claim your limbs,
then shall you truly dance.

—Kahlil Gibran

Find out what the dying person wants and, if possible, meet his or her wishes. If you don't feel comfortable with these wishes—for example, the dying person wants cremation and you find it horrifying—discuss your feelings with him or her. Unnecessary pain is caused after a death if we feel torn between wanting to follow a loved one's wishes and our distaste for their choice. Probably no dying loved one would want additional pain for you if they were aware of your feelings. As we become more comfortable talking about dying and its aftermath, hopefully more dying people will say, "I prefer _________, and I want you to do what feels best to you at the time."

The choices for disposal of the body are cremation, burial, or bequeathal to science.

Unless you plan to bury the body yourself, I suggest you check first with a memorial society, a local volunteer-run branch of the Funeral Consumers Alliance (FCA). These groups help members make prearrangements for a simple, economical burial. Because they're nonprofit, they'll give you straight information about legal requirements, costs, and arrangements. There are now about two hundred memorial societies in the United States and Canada. Membership runs fifteen to thirty dollars, and anyone can join. If you're quoted a higher membership price, it's probably not a real memorial society.

Memorial societies do what we often don't: shop around and compare services and prices. They generally act in an advisory capacity, not offering services themselves but providing information about local services. In my experience they're fine people who know what's happening in the community and are very helpful.

To find one, look in the white pages of your telephone book under "memorial society" or "funeral society." If you don't find a listing, call FCA at 1–800–765–0107 or locate them on the internet at www.funerals.org.

One of the finest books about death and dying is Ernest Morgan's *A Manual of Death Education and Simple Burial,* which is available from memorial societies or from Amazon.com.

Cremation

Burning a body until only ashes remain is a simple, clean, economical way of returning earth to earth. Cremation was the preferred method of disposing of a body for 36 percent of Americans in 2008 and is expected to rise to about 46 percent by 2015.[1] Actual cremation costs about $150 to $250. You can take the body to a crematory yourself or have a funeral home take it.

Most people prefer to have a funeral home make cremation arrangements. If that's your choice and you want to keep expenses down, call all the funeral homes in your area and ask for the price of "direct cremation with a minimum alternative container." Prices vary widely, from $500 to $2,000. "Direct cremation," or "direct disposal," includes picking up the body, refrigerating it for the forty-eight-hour waiting period required by law, doing the paperwork, having the body cremated, and returning the ashes to you. It does not include a service, urn, or niche in the cemetery. If you've made an arrangement with a funeral home, call them when you want the body removed.

Crematories require a suitable container for the body, such as a simple wood or heavy cardboard box. A casket and embalming are not legally required for cremation. The funeral home will give you the ashes in a cardboard box. You can scatter them when you choose, keep them at home, or in a cemetery niche, which may be expensive. Scattering the ashes helps us focus on a living spirit instead of on a cocoon. If you live in California, Indiana, Alaska, or Washington, check with your county coroner about limitations on scattering ashes.

Overseeing a cremation yourself is hard work when you're emotionally and/or physically exhausted, and it can be very satisfying. Anybody can take a body to a crematory without the services of a funeral director as long as the legal requirements are met. These include getting the death certificate, transit permit, authorization to cremate, filing with any other authorities, refrigerating the body for forty-eight hours at the crematory or funeral home, and a proper body container. You can build your own wood box or buy a cardboard one from the crematory.

If you choose to handle arrangements yourself, check with the coroner or medical examiner to determine exact legal requirements where the death takes place. You may run into opposition along the way, not because what you're doing is illegal but because it's unusual. Many funeral directors are fine, responsible people.

A friend, Bix Cramer, whom I consider Germany's greatest product beside Goethe and Volkswagens, was married to an American painter. After he died at home, she looked in the Austin, Texas, yellow pages to find a mortuary. She asked the director of the King of Tears Mortuary (I swear I didn't make up that name) for the cheapest cremation. She said, "The staff was great. They didn't try to sell me extra stuff, and the price was about $1,200." The obituary for the newspaper, which she wrote, said, "Martin S. Cramer was brought into this world on October 28, 1941, without his knowledge and consent. He died against his will on July 21, 1996..."

Earth Burial

In our country, earth burial is the most common form of disposing of a body. It has become extremely costly unless you live in a state that permits burial on private property, or the person is eligible to be buried in a National Cemetery. (See the section in chapter 4, "Veterans Administration" for eligibility.)

If your state permits burial on private property, it can be very satisfying to do the burial yourself. Plan ahead: You will need to present the death certificate to the local registrar of vital statistics, or appropriate agency, to obtain a burial or transit permit. A professional carpenter or friend can build the coffin. For an adult, the box should be six inches to one foot longer than the person, about one to one and one-half feet deep, and two feet to three feet wide. It should have a separate top that can be put on later. Line the box and decorate the outside if you wish. Use the box to transport the body to the chosen burial place, where you'll probably want to have a service. For digging, you need shovels, picks, and a strong back and/or a backhoe.

Home burials cost almost nothing. John's burial cost $150. This included two trees to start the orchard and food and drink for the celebration. Mary's funeral cost $44, which included wood for the coffin, gasoline for two trucks, and beer for the diggers. My parents' funerals were handled by a funeral home and, although simple, were quite expensive.

If the laws in your state don't permit burial on private property or you don't want to handle arrangements yourself, you'll need to make them, if you haven't already, with a funeral home and cemetery. Added to the cost of funeral home services are cemetery expenses. They include buying a plot, digging the hole and closing it, a concrete liner or vault, and a simple grave marker and can cost from $500 to thousands of dollars.

Most cemeteries require a casket to be placed in a concrete liner or a vault to prevent the ground above the grave from sinking. Sometimes moisture-proof vaults are recommended as a way to preserve the body. A body in a $15,000 vault will decay just like one in a concrete liner or a blanket, as Native Americans traditionally use—perhaps faster.

FUNERAL HOMES

The dollars spent for a funeral don't say anything.

—A funeral director

In 2006, the National Funeral Directors Association reported that the average American funeral cost $7,323.[2] Not included in this cost are cemetery fees. By now, the costs are higher.

After a home and car, a funeral is the third largest purchase most Americans make. Unlike for the first two major purchases, we don't shop around when it comes to funerals. We usually use a funeral home because "My family's always used them." The funeral industry took advantage of our vulnerability and failure to comparison shop and took us for a financial ride. They're not solely responsible; we played victims.

In the past, funeral industry practices got so outrageous that the Federal Trade Commission in 1984 stepped in and passed the Funeral Rule. This law requires, among other things, that funeral homes provide prices of individual services over the telephone. They are also required to give you a written price list of goods and services when you visit to inquire about services. The law makes it possible for you to buy individual items as well as package services and goods.

If you're not emotionally up to comparison shopping, ask someone to call for you and then make your choices. There's wide disparity in prices.

The Funeral Rule makes it illegal for funeral homes to represent to you that embalming is a legal requirement when it's not. In most places embalming is not required unless a body is to be transported across state lines, preserved beyond a certain time limit, or the death was caused by a communicable disease. Embalming is not a religious requirement. It's expressly forbidden, and considered a desecration of the body, by the Jewish Orthodox faith.

Instead of being embalmed, a body can be refrigerated until a service, burial, or cremation. To rationalize embalming, funeral directors sometimes say that viewing the body aids families in their grieving process. It's true that viewing the body is important; it seems to cauterize the emotional wound. But, even in a sudden death, the body may be viewed on the spot or in the hospital emergency room. In a home death, you've had time to experience the physical reality of death and there's usually no need for "viewing the body." If there is a need, it can be viewed refrigerated.

Caskets are generally the most expensive funeral item. No state law has explicit casket requirements. Consider having a service without a casket, without the body present, or, if you want it present, consider a simple wood box or cardboard container. Don't let funeral home personnel talk you into a "protective seal" on a coffin to preserve the body. It's totally unnecessary.

The least expensive casket will probably not be on display in the funeral home showroom because they get a commission on caskets. Feel free to ask to see it. Don't believe anyone who tells you a $150 casket doesn't show the respect of a $3,000 one. Respect is an attitude, not a coffin. The dying person may already have expressed definite preferences on this subject.

A fancy funeral or casket is not an effective way to deal with grief or guilt. If you like a big show, why not have a super memorial party? Or, you might want to give the money you'd have spent to a person or group who needs it, perhaps one favored by the person who died. Don't be manipulated into spending more on a funeral than you want. Statements such as "He deserves the best," "This is the last thing you can do for your mother," "That's the welfare funeral," or "Spend enough to do the deceased credit" are overt manipulation.

What about getting a pine coffin and painting it yourself and/or with family and friends? Two resources for beautiful finished coffins are www.mainecottagegarden.com and www.trappistcaskets.com.

GREEN BURIALS

Green cemeteries were reestablished in 1993 in England where there are now over two hundred. In the United States, as "going green" has become a focus for us, many people are looking for environmentally friendly alternatives to expensive polluting burials, and even to cremation. A number of states already have laws permitting simple natural burial and many others are considering them.

What's new in funerals is as old as humankind. After death, the deceased's remains are wrapped in a cotton shroud or wool blanket and placed directly in the earth. Or, sometimes a simple biodegradable wood box, a basket, or even a recycled paper casket. Native plants, flowers, and shrubs are planted over the body. Land stewardship and restoration are an important aspect of green burials. The burial site is marked with a small, flat stone or can be located by global positioning system (GPS) coordinates.

A wealth of information about green funerals is the Green Burial Council, www.greenburialcouncil.org. Others that provide information as well as products are www.naturalburialcompany.com and www.thegreenfuneralsite.com. For people who prefer cremation and love the ocean, check out www.eternalreefs.com, which offers underwater burial at sea in artificial reefs.

John and Mary's green funerals were deeply satisfying.

BEQUEATHAL OF A BODY

Bequeathal of the body to science is another way to dispose of a cocoon. Make arrangements, if possible, before the death, with your state organ procurement organization, which you can locate online at OrganDonor.gov or through a medical school.

Some medical schools have more bodies than they need and others not enough. They'll generally pick up the body. If you live a great distance from the school, however, you may have to pay part of the transportation costs. Ask them while you're on the phone. Their release form includes what you want done with the body afterward.

RITUALS AND CELEBRATIONS

A ritual or celebration facilitates the process of grieving by allowing family and friends to express their love for the living spirit and for each other.

Leaving a physical vehicle, the body, is an important rite of passage for both the person doing it and for the family and friends. A ritual marking this change helps us express our sadness and loss with others before we face our changed reality, sometimes seemingly alone.

A memorial service is a service generally held two or three days after the death without the body present. In a funeral service, the body is present in a casket. A committal service is a brief service held at a graveside, in the chapel of a crematory, or wherever the ashes are scattered.

Allow a celebration to grow in whatever way feels appropriate for you. Choose a place that's meaningful—indoors or out in nature. Does it matter if the body is present or not? Do you, the people involved, want to speak about your feelings? Would you rather be silent? Do you want someone to lead the ceremony, or can each person share in their own way? Do you want clergy, or do you want to be your own minister and celebrants? Do you want flowers, music, or poetry? Do you want to share food or dancing or song? What about a prayer circle, or a hug or holding circle? Even digging can be part of the ritual.

The ritual you create can be a celebration of life. We can celebrate the life completed, and through it, all of life. We can celebrate love. We can celebrate the joy of sharing times together. We can share love and support for each other, and perhaps anger that we're left to take care of daily business.

Jewish *shivas,* Irish and Polish wakes, and Hispanic *veladas* (candlelight watches) have long been useful forms for exploring and sharing loss and renewing old relationships.

You might use an old form or create a new one.

In a ritual, I believe we need to focus on releasing the soul even if it is difficult for us. If we cling to it, the soul's love for us makes it difficult for it to move away from family, friends, and the familiar physical world and on to its new life.

We're accustomed to thinking there is nothing further we can do for someone after he or she dies. We speak at our services as if they aren't there. I believe they are there and that we can still help. We can talk with the person, let them know we're okay, and encourage them to go free. We can offer prayers of thanksgiving for life that never ends, and we can continue to share our hearts.

Working with Clergy

If your spiritual understanding and practices have been related to a particular faith community, you may want to ask your minister, rabbi, or priest for helping in planning a service. The clergy have shared their knowledge and compassion many times with dying people and their families. They do have a commitment to do things in the manner prescribed by their particular faith. Check within yourself to see if their suggestions meet the earlier wishes of the person as well as your own sense of rightness. Everyone has equal access to God.

What to Wear

What to wear for a funeral is still an issue for many people. You might think, "Darn, I don't have a black dress or suit. Will navy blue do?"

I don't happen to like wearing black. It makes me feel locked in, constricted. Wearing black forms a shield around the body that retards energy going in or out and protects us when we're emotionally weak. But the price of this protection is high. Black locks in energy, including sadness, grief, and love. In countries where it's the custom to wear black for a long mourning period, holding in feelings frequently becomes a way of life. In my view, wearing black is like a heavy casket: it keeps things in. Can you remember anyone wearing black in all those paintings of the death of Jesus Christ? No, they wore white or light colors. White is expansive and reflects energy. I suggest wearing a color you like or one you know the butterfly liked.

We can reflect the rainbow. Respect is an attitude, not a color.

A LIFE CELEBRATION TO SHARE LATER

Death is not extinguishing the light
but putting out the candle because the dawn has come.
—Rabindranath Tagore

The blessing of having shared time and love with someone doesn't end just because they're no longer here in a body.

In the months to come, you might want to create something to celebrate their life, and your life: a garden, an orchard, a carved cross, or whatever. Making a card or writing a story or poem can be a healing way to share someone's movement from life to life, particularly with friends who weren't present for the death or burial. Months after John died, an artist friend hauled a rock down off a mesa, carved it, and set it on John's grave.

Many people expect the anniversary of physical death or the person's birthday to be a day of sadness. If we expect them to be sad, they will be. However, we can make them days to celebrate the joy of having loved them. Consider putting flowers in your living room that you might have put on the grave to remind you of that joy.

I was deeply moved by the celebration for a woman I never met: Jean Lake.

Before she died of cancer, Jean dreamed of publishing a book of her paintings of rural life in Alabama and simple sayings she'd found helpful in her life. One day after she died, one of her young children was talking with a family friend and mentioned her mother's dream. The dream touched her friend's heart. She resolved to publish the book, whatever it took, and give the proceeds for an art scholarship at a local college. In the process of completing the book, *Seeds to Sow* (Troy State University Press), she married her friend's husband. So, the dream of the first wife was carried out by the second wife. And the story didn't end with the publication of the book. Now an annual art festival, the Troyfest, in honor of Jean Lake, is the centerpiece of their town's cultural life.

CELEBRATING MY MOTHER'S LIFE

One joy scatters a hundred griefs.

—Chinese proverb

Sometimes your joy is the source of your smile,
but sometimes your smile can be the source of your joy.

—Theodore Roethke

I'd like to share the story of how I celebrated my mother's life and eased my sense of loss.

About a year before Mom died, I'd had a dream in Spanish in which I heard, "When your mother dies, go to Monte Alban and your tears will be changed into joy...*que sus lagrimas serian cambiados por la alegria.*" Having lived in Mexico, I was vaguely aware that Monte Alban was located in the south, somewhere near Oaxaca. But I didn't know if it was a Mayan ruin or a Catholic monastery, or perhaps both.

Two days after the funeral, I flew to Oaxaca. I'd only have one full day there before I had to be back on Kaua'i. Since Hurricane Iniki had devastated my island home, I'd been working as regional coordinator for a FEMA-funded mental health recovery program.

I quickly located a red-tile-roofed colonial *posada,* or hotel, not far from the main plaza. I dumped my bags in the room without unpacking and walked on cobblestoned streets to the open-air market. Gleefully sucking on a *Granada China,* a burgundy-colored, papery-skinned passion fruit, I wandered through a maze of flower stalls. I treated myself to a bouquet of white flowers—baby's breath, exquisitely fragrant tuberoses, and calla lilies—so huge that walking back to the hotel, I couldn't see my feet.

After banking my room with the flowers, I rang up the concierge. "Where and what is Monte Alban? I have to go there."

He replied, "It's a group of pyramids about a half hour from here by car. I can arrange a driver for tomorrow."

That night, lying alone in a hotel bed like a ceremonial altar, surrounded by the flowers, I prayed, "God, please help me to celebrate Mom's life and her death."

The next day *just happened to be* the Fiesta of the Virgin of Guadalupe, one of Mexico's most joyful celebrations. Thousands of people packed the plaza to celebrate Don Diego's visions of the Virgin.

Surrounded by colonial cathedrals, enormous green shade trees, and outdoor cafés, the plaza was filled with *mariachis,* red and pink helium balloons, and the smells of roast pork, *carnitas,* and frying doughnuts. Hundreds of babies and children were dressed like Don Diego in sombreros and red kerchiefs with little black moustaches painted on cherubic brown faces. Speaking Spanish with smiling parents holding up their children for me to admire, my heart smiled and my mouth couldn't help but follow suit.

Wandering away from the noisy, pungent gaiety of the central plaza, through quieter cobblestone streets and smaller plazas bordered by cathedrals, I encountered a roadside market selling typical indigenous clothing. My eyes riveted on a red *huipil,* a handwoven dress worn by Zapotec women. "This would be the perfect Christmas dress to wear each year to celebrate Mom's life," I thought. For my budget, even with shrewd bargaining, the price was too high.

Wandering on to the Plaza de Santo Domingo, I fell into conversation with *campesinos* planting hundreds of red, pink, and white poinsettias. The Mexican government, sensitive to the value of beauty, each year hires people to plant hundreds of thousands of poinsettias in plazas all over the country. As I admired the planters' work, the conversation turned to the reason for my visit to Oaxaca. "I've come to celebrate my mother's life and her death." I mentioned the red dress and wanting it to celebrate her life. Two women volunteered to go buy the dress. We assumed, because they were *Indios,* they could purchase it for less. When they returned empty-handed, reporting they'd been asked an even higher price, we laughed and laughed.

On my return to the hotel, the driver was waiting to take me to Monte Alban. He explained that it had been a ceremonial center used by Olmec, Zapotec, and Mixtec Indians.

The sky was every imaginable color of blue feathered with white clouds as the van labored up the narrow, twisting road toward the ancient spiritual gathering place. Leaving below the confusion, chatter, commerce, and dust of the plains, I felt excited, yet peaceful. The summit of Monte Alban looked as if a giant cleaver had sliced off the top of the mountain. In its place, ancient peoples had covered the plateau with towering stone pyramids in alignment with the planets and stars, to honor the sun, moon, Jaguar God, and Quetzacoatl, the plumed serpent.

Atop the plateau, standing alone in the wind, listening to silence, I felt as if I were perched on a giant condor's nest. Monte Alban is the exact epicenter of a vast, pale apple-green valley dotted with villages and encircled by distant mountains now muted in haze. Closing my eyes, I could see the unadorned pyramids in their splendor of long ago—plastered in brilliant white, decorated in gold, hot pink, and turquoise. I felt happy and totally alive.

After a while, I wandered to the edge of the plateau and sat down on a pile of dirt and unsorted pyramid rubble. In silence, broken only by the wind, I somehow knew that Mom and I had been here before. Together in another time or level of reality...and it had been a happy one.

Mom's spirit felt present. Silently, I said to her, "Mom, the only thing that bothered me about your twelve-year journey with illness was why someone as loving and conscious as you had to suffer so much." Clearly, I heard her say, "I'd lost my faith, Deborah. The whole purpose of my life was to get it back."

As she spoke, I felt lighter; years of real, yet invisible, weight lifted off me. In an instant confusion vanished and it was clear that regaining her faith was worth whatever we'd gone through together. Tears of elation ran down my face. "Mom, you did it," I said. "You did it."

Standing tall and free in the wind, high atop Monte Alban, I knew that although my physical parents were gone from the earth, the ongoing spiritual legacy of my birth mother was surrender and faith.

Joy filled every cell of my being until there was no "I" separate from anything in the universe.

Weeping may endure for a night, but joy cometh in the morning.

—Psalm 30:5

15

GRIEVING

Perhaps the most important reason for 'lamenting' is that it helps us to realize our oneness with all things, to know that all things are our relatives...

—Black Elk

If you know in your heart that your loved one is alive although alive in a different way, you may feel joy as well as sadness. Allow joy. Allow relief. If you hurt, you need to express the pain so you don't suffer later.

Allow yourself to grieve. Allow your grief to express in whatever way feels right to you. Grieving is the way we heal the loss we feel for someone we love. If you have grieved throughout this dying journey and/or if the relationship with the person wasn't central to your life, you may not feel sad. That's fine. No need to pretend to grieve.

If you hurt, know that you're not crazy. A deep, bursting sorrow is one reflection of the value in your life of this close relationship. You may feel things similar to those the person experienced: denial, isolation, guilt, anger, bargaining, depression, and acceptance.

Cry those oceans if they're there. Yell. Be sad, be lonely, be helpless, be out of control, be angry. Move your body. Don't let anyone tell you to be quieter; they can do it their way when it's their turn to grieve. Yell at "John the Bastard" for leaving you. Yell at "God the Merciless" for taking your child. Let it spill out of all the nooks and crannies of your being. Cry for all those things you didn't cry about in the past. Clean out old sadness.

At some point, the emptiness will come. Know this space. It may be with you for a time and it may be one of the most important spaces in your life. It's in this quiet after the outward grieving that the seeds for your new life begin to grow. Some people call this emptiness the "dark night of the soul." You've let go of something precious and familiar, and what will give your life meaning in the future is not yet known. It takes a lot of courage to be alive in this emptiness. Just be with it. Pay attention to what is trying to grow: new qualities or ways of being, new ideas about life, work, whatever.

There's a Zen saying, "You can't fill a teacup that is already full." If we allow the emptiness, we can move to a new fullness.

As you begin to understand what is trying to grow, and if you're willing, nourish these tiny seedlings. If you panic, you may crush little new beginnings. A lot of people panic. I have. Because this emptiness is often unknown and frightening, we rush to fill the void with activity or suffering—perhaps the closest, most familiar thing at this moment. Maybe we say to ourselves, "Better to feel something, even if it's suffering, than nothing at all." It's true that a vacuum looks to be filled; however, we have a choice what we fill it with. We have a choice! You can use this quiet space instead of it using you. Catch up on sleep, eat balanced meals, pray, meditate, take long walks, work in the garden. Prepare your soil. If possible, if the death was someone very close to you, put off major decisions for at least a year.

When our hearts break, they break open, making more room for everybody and everything: more love, more joy, more compassion. We can stay open to the loneliness and pain, knowing it's moving us to a new fullness. Or we can shut down. A heart that has broken open doesn't close unless we close it. We make the choice.

Part of grieving is fear. We're afraid we've lost our love, that somehow it's gone with the physical body of the person. But without the soul that shone through that person, we probably wouldn't have loved him or her in the first place, and the soul is not gone. We don't have to stop thinking about or stop loving the person. I believe it's inaccurate to assume that the *object* of our love is our love. We are love, so we can never lose it.

We can expand our love, which may recently have been focused almost exclusively on one person, to include more and more people. Give your love to yourself. Loving yourself is the greatest gift you can give to the people you love, present in a body or not. When you feel able, give love to the people around you. If there aren't any, find new people and situations in which you can share love. When you give it away, it always returns to you increased.

If we don't express our feelings, including our love, we feel depressed. Our love backs up on us and poisons our lives instead of illuminating them. I don't remember feeling depressed around the people I love while they were dying. Depression often comes afterward, when suddenly there's no longer a clear focus for our love and energy, no one to care for, no obvious way of expressing our love.

The solution to depression caused by trapped love is to find new ways to express it, which is not too difficult really. It's needed everywhere. The teenager who bags your groceries needs it, your neighbors need it, babies need it, old people need it, prisoners need it, the animals at the local shelter need it. Don't be put off if they're not yet skilled receivers of love; perhaps you know what that's like yourself.

I've observed, and experienced, two kinds of grieving: grieving for cleansing and healing, and grieving as a habit of suffering. The first is essential for growth; the second offers no movement. It's like treading water. Who wants to tread water for the rest of their lives? It's tiring—and boring. Cleansing and healing provide space for delicate, and perhaps exciting, new growth.

The barn's burned down,
Now I can see the moon.

—Masahide
Japanese poet

If you feel stuck in suffering, get help. Find a friend or counselor. Finding someone who works with techniques that focus on releasing stuck feelings may be useful. Some cultures meet the need for grieving with wailing, dancing, chanting—all ways of releasing pent-up energies. However, in our culture we tend to find such releases embarrassing, so sometimes we need counselors. We probably won't need them anymore when we stop making judgments against our feelings and instead start appreciating the help expressing them gives us in adjusting to life's great changes.

Avoid drugs and alcohol. They may temporarily ease your pain but will delay or stop the necessary grieving process. If you're alone at home, have already let out all your tears, and the pain still feels too heavy, send love to the part of you that hurts. Try compressing time. Imagine yourself a year from now. How are you feeling? Is there more space around the pain? Write your feelings on paper.

Talk, perhaps out loud, to the person you're missing. She or he can still hear you. A 2005 Gallup Poll reported that 21 percent of Americans believe we can communicate with people after their death.[1] So, if you do, you're not crazy, or else you've got a lot of company. You might want to call Unity Prayer at 1-800-669-7729.

To quote American writer Samuel Coleridge, "Look for the rainbow, that gracious thing made up of tears and light." There's a Persian proverb that says, "When it's dark, you can see the stars." Would it help to take a chair outside at night and watch the stars?

During your grieving, allow friends the opportunity to share with you. Improve your ability to receive gracefully and allow friends to experience the joy of giving. They'll feel privileged that you chose to talk with them about your feelings about the person you love. Sometimes they can help you recognize the new seeds sprouting. And they can hold you when you need it. Ask. Often, friends want to share their love and don't know how. Tell them what you need. It's after the first month or first year, when the shock and numbness begin to wear off, that we particularly need their support.

In the jungles of Mexico they have a useful custom. After someone dies, each person who comes to the funeral or to visit asks the mourner to recount the story of how the death happened. The visitors probably already know, but the point is to keep the mourner repeating and repeating the story until the shock lessens and he or she begins to accept what's happened. Friends can do the same for us: listen and listen and listen. Share your story. It will help you, and others will benefit as well.

In addition to sharing with friends, it's healing to share with people who've had a similar experience. All hospice programs have bereavement support groups. If you did not participate in a hospice program, to locate a support group, call your church or the social service office of a hospital. If your child died, as mentioned earlier, Compassionate Friends, a national organization with about 500 local support groups, can help you locate a group in your area. Again, see appendix D for a parent's suggestion on healing your grief by writing your child's story.

Books with practical ideas to help us mend an injured or broken heart can also be helpful. Dr. Roberta Temes in *Living with an Empty Chair: A Guide Through Grief* describes our response to loss in terms of numbness, disorganization, and reorganization. I recommend *How to Survive the Loss of Love* by McWilliams (Bantam Books); *Don't Take My Grief Away* by Doug Manning (Harper and Row); and *The Bereaved Parent* by Harriet Schiff (Penguin Books).

If you want a reminder about joy, I highly recommend *To Hear the Angels Sing* by Dorothy Maclean (Lorian Press) and my favorite book, *Emmanuel's Book,* compiled by Pat Rodegast (Friends Press).

Take time to appreciate yourself. You are the same person who began this experience and at the same time, you aren't. You have changed and grown in immeasurable ways.

In case it happens to slip your mind, remember: spring has always come and it always will.

Death is nothing at all. I have only slipped away into the next room. I am I and you are you: Whatever we were to each other, that we are still. Call me by my old familiar name. Speak to me in the easy way you always used. Put no difference into your tone; wear no forced air of solemnity or sorrow. Laugh as we always laughed at the little jokes we enjoyed together. Play, smile, think of me, pray for me. Let my name be ever the household word that it always was. Let it be spoken without effort, without the ghost of a shadow on it.
Life means all that it ever meant.
It is the same as it ever was; there is absolute unbroken continuity. What is death but a negligible accident?
I am waiting for you, for an interval, somewhere very near, just around the corner. All is well.

—Canon Scott Holland
Facts of the Faith

16

LIFE AFTER DEATH

Souls are poured from one into another of different kinds of bodies of the world.

—Jesus Christ
Gnostic Gospels: Pistis Sophia

People sleep and when they die they awake.

—Mohammad

Your own heart is the best source of knowing about life after death. I can share with you my reality and how I arrived at it. I can tell you about recent studies and writings across the ages. For example, a 2007 article in the AARP magazine reported that 73 percent of Americans over fifty believe in life after death.[1] But, all of these are just footnotes to your own knowing.

If you're willing, try this:

Find a quiet place and close your eyes. Breathe gently inside and let go of any ideas you have about life after death. Become empty. If thoughts come up, don't get caught up in them; just watch them. Breathe into your heart area and from this place ask for guidance. Ask if death exists. Ask if we're born again and again. Trust what you hear, especially if it's a calm, gentle inner voice. If nothing comes, that's okay too.

Working with dying people, I've found that most have had hints or visions that life continues and/or that they've lived before and will again. When they felt that I wouldn't judge them crazy or senile, many dying people shared experiences they'd not shared before. We learn a lot about our common human experience when people feel free to share their experiences without fear of being ridiculed.

Mark Twain said, "I've been born more times than anybody except Krishna." And Voltaire said, "It is not more surprising to be born twice than once; everything in nature is resurrection."

One of the glorious things about being alive in our time is that mystics and scientists are finally beginning to say the same things. Mystics have always believed life continues after death. Some scientists are beginning to say, "Well, maybe." To mystics, the one family of humankind has always been a reality. Biochemists at the University of California were some of the first scientists to prove genetically that all the humans alive today had the same mother. Their study used a part of the cell inherited only from the mother. More recently, the Genographic Project of the National Geographic Society widely disseminated the news that everyone living today carries the genes of "Scientific Adam," our original father, who lived some 60,000 years ago in Africa.[2] We're beginning to realize that the mystic and scientific paths are both valid ways to approach truth.

Dr. Kübler-Ross said, "I don't have a shadow of doubt death as an end doesn't really exist...If they hang me up by my toes, I won't stop exploring life after death."

Raymond Moody, MD, in his popular book *Life After Life,* reports the experience of people who "officially died" and were resuscitated. Since his book, numerous books and articles on near-death experiences, NDEs, have been published. Many are by medical doctors who received firsthand reports from patients and by ordinary people who've had the experience themselves.

What Dr. Moody reports basically agrees with what dying people have told me. From his interviews with people who died and were resuscitated, he reports the following:

- When the "officially dead" persons heard someone say they were dead, they felt surprised and afraid.
- After the initial fear, they felt incredibly peaceful.
- Some reported hearing noises: buzzing, ringing, roaring, chimes, or bells.
- Most experienced a dark space, often described as a tunnel, which they moved through quickly.
- Many then experienced being outside of their bodies and looking down, surprised at the efforts being made to revive them. Vision and hearing seemed enhanced.
- Most reported reunions with relatives and friends who'd died earlier, who acted sort of as a greeting committee.
- Nearly all experienced a beautiful luminous light or "light being" who felt enormously loving. The identification of this light being was determined by their experience before death. (Dr. Karlis Osis and Erlendur Haraldson made a cross-cultural study between the United States and India. They found that Christians interpreted the light being as Christ and Hindus interpreted it as a Hindu deity. Both Asians and Americans saw the dark passage, brilliant light, and "dead" relatives.)
- The light being often suggested that the person review their life. No one reported feeling this was punitive, only instructive.
- The person reached a barrier or limit where they felt they must choose whether or not to return to life. Most found "being dead" so beautiful that returning was a hard decision. Many decided to return only because of their great love for their children or spouse.
- After the experience, most felt they wouldn't be afraid to die again. And their experience of life was greatly enhanced.

What about heaven and hell? Each of us defines them in our own way. To me, they're states of consciousness rather than places. Heaven is consciousness of union with everything, with God. Hell is consciousness of separation. Heaven is remembering who we are. Hell is forgetting: believing we're separate and alone. Heaven is love. Hell is fear.

If there is only one time-space, then after we die we all go to the same "place." If we got what we deserved based on some of our unkind behavior in life, there probably would be a hell. I believe we get what we deserve based on who we most profoundly are, no matter what the outward appearances: love. And love is the reward for love. So I believe in a heaven, a "place" of love, after physical death.

I also believe as surely as hell has existed on earth, so does heaven exist on earth. To experience heaven on earth, we have to heal the eye of the heart so we see life through the lens of love instead of the lens of fear. Then we see the beauty, courage, and nobility of our human family and the exquisite natural beauty of the earth. When we're in love, we experience heaven on earth. That's why we long for that experience. Through our much-disparaged rose-colored glasses, we see the truth. Heaven is already on earth. We don't have to wait until we die to experience it.

To me, hell is all the things we create when we see life though the lens of fear. Hell is punishment. If life is a school for remembering love, as I like to think, would God punish us because we stumble and fall? It seems unlikely to me. I imagine that each time we fall, the God in us picks us up, dusts us off, says, "I love you," and we start again. No one punishes us except ourselves.

Evidently, after we die, we review our lives so we can learn from our experience. Perhaps this review is what some call hell or purgatory. Reexperiencing some of the unloving things we've done can be awful. Once, my whole life flashed before me, and I felt enormous pain just witnessing myself turning my back on someone whose eyes were asking me for love or help. I hate to think how I'd have felt if I'd killed someone. But perhaps in terms of unconditional love, killing someone physically and killing someone emotionally by withholding love are of equal weight.

What about sin and evil? To me, they're energy we haven't looked into deeply enough to fully understand. Sin and evil are a lack of love. So they are healed by love, not punishment, which is just more lack of love. At times, we may have to physically segregate someone so they won't hurt us while they're learning to love. However, prisons won't be effective rehabilitation centers until they teach people to love.

Punishment is a form of manipulation. It's a way to control people with fear. Perhaps hell—major punishment—was invented so some groups could control their members with fear. Many organized religions suggest that *their* way is the only way to God. Follow instructions or be punished! This is not to deny the beauty of organized religions, but only to point out that they are made up of people like you and me who have free will and are, therefore, fallible.

I believe we can't give the responsibility for our relationship with God, with life, to anyone else. We are each ultimately responsible.

Until the Second Council of Constantinople in A.D. 553, reincarnation, which teaches that we're responsible for our thoughts and behavior, was included in the Bible. Jesus himself indicated his belief in reincarnation when he said that John the Baptist was Elijah, the dead prophet returned (Matthew 11:14). Also, Jesus was an Essene, and they believed in reincarnation.

For more than five hundred years, reincarnation, "the mystical doctrine," was widely accepted by Christians, including the most eminent church fathers. The Council, presided

It is the secret of the world that all things subsist and do not die, but only retire a little from sight and afterwards return again. Nothing is dead, men feign themselves dead, and endure mock funerals...and there they stand looking out of the window, sound and well, in some strange new disguise.

—Ralph Waldo Emerson

over by the Emperor Augustinian, declared it heresy.[3] They called it "the mythical doctrine" and deleted it from the Bible by a vote of three to two. Perhaps it was politically expedient for the Church for people not to know that they had more than one chance to get to heaven, or that eventually everyone gets there no matter what their religious path.[4] Reincarnation is still found in the writings of St. Augustine, a man who inspires both Catholics and non-Catholics.

The fundamental premise of reincarnation is that everyone is in the process of returning home to God or growing to godhood. And we are born again and again until we reach that union. Each soul is created equal to every other soul. Each soul has free will to remember its true nature in its *own* way and its *own* time. No time or way is better than another. The paths home are as many as the people on the earth. Nothing can stop our homeward journey. Any delays we might experience are just opportunities to deepen our understanding.

Reincarnation teaches that we choose when and to whom we will be born. We choose our parents, the ones most suitable to provide the environment we need to complete any unlearned lessons. As a soul, we enter the physical child conceived by the chosen parents. We reincarnate in groups, so we see again and again people we've loved and helped as well and those we've hated and hurt. According to this belief system, our coming together as families and friends is no accident.

We also choose when we will die. When the soul sees that the body is no longer in condition to support our continued learning, it gives a signal for the dying process to begin. Sometimes the soul leaves the body before the body stops functioning. This may explain a feeling commonly reported by people on deathbed watches: they sense the person has already gone.

According to the belief of reincarnation, we create, allow, or tolerate everything we experience in our lives in order to help us learn, or remember. We don't always get what we *consciously* want in life; we get what we believe or what we fear. No one is a victim. Assuming we're victims is a way we avoid taking responsibility for what we create. Once we remember who we really are and become responsible co-creators, we aren't born again—unless we choose to return to serve our fellow human beings.

"Whatsoever a man sows, that shall he also reap" (Galatians 6:7). The cause and effect of our actions is sometimes called the Law of Karma. The law is simply a description of how energy works. Plant a carrot; reap a carrot. Give love, receive love. Karma may also be understood as our unlearned lessons and/or as judgments we make that keep us feeling separate.

Karma means we're responsible and accountable for all past choices and actions no matter how small. We reap the blessings and the teachings. Being sick, having a car accident, or going to jail are not punishment or "bad karma." They are opportunities we've created to help us remember or learn so we can change our lives and live more joyfully.

There's also group karma. I believe, for example, it's the karma of the human race and individuals to learn to live together in peace. World War II, for example, was a reminder we created that we weren't doing too well. It was group karma, but no one chose to be alive at that time who didn't have the individual karma to learn from it.

Unconditional love doesn't create karma. If in any situation my intention was love, I am responsible for love. If hate was my intention, I'm responsible for hate, and karma is created. "Working out karma"—being responsible for what we feel, think, say, and do—teaches love and compassion. It helps us move beyond separation to the truth of unity.

Unconditional love transcends karma. Another way of saying that is "Divine will transcends the cause and effect of human will." Sometimes this is called the Law of Grace. Grace is the teaching of compassion that Jesus Christ added to the older Hindu and Buddhist teaching of divine justice, karma.

For example, if I become a different person from the one I was when I created the karma (by changing, transforming, repenting, or re-thinking), I'm free of it. Karma is education, not punishment, and I've learned my lesson.

Justice is the great teaching of the mind; love, compassion, and freedom are the perhaps greater teachings of the heart.

Unconditional love heals, completes, and finishes karma. At any time we can break the cycle of birth, death, and rebirth by loving unconditionally. It may take many lifetimes. Or, it's possible for you and me to do it right now.

In a very real sense, helping others love the God within them is helping ourselves, for as John Donne famously said, "No man is an island...(each) is a piece of the continent, a part of the main...any man's death diminishes me, because I am involved in mankind, and therefore never send to know for whom the bell tolls. It tolls for you."

Perhaps our work is to love, to serve, and to remember.

When we see all of nature working in cycles, I often wonder why we don't envision the same for ourselves. Is it arrogance, or is it fear that we'll lose our individuality, our specialness, if we're part of some larger whole? Are we confusing uniformity with unity? Each flower, tree, sunset, and human being gives its unique gift to the whole. We see a seed planted, growing to maturity, bearing fruit, decaying, dying, and releasing seeds that sprout anew. Over and over we see the cycle of birth, death, and rebirth.

Are we not too part of the cyclical process of nature? Does not the seed-core in us continue to grow after our bodies die?

❧

I'd like to share with you how my understanding of the continuity of life grew.

As a child when I was still closely connected to my heart-knowing, I knew that life didn't end. But the adults around me said it ended with death, and they were bigger than me and I wanted their approval. (Interestingly, children up to five years old believe death is reversible.)[5] It didn't make sense to me that we came into the world, did this little dance, and were snuffed out.

I heard a lot of talk about justice, loving our brothers, freedom, and perfection that didn't make sense in terms of what I saw around me. "Why are they starving?" "Why was their son killed in an accident?" "Why are we so lucky?" "Why is his wife so mean to him?" "Why is she dying of cancer? She's such a good person."

It seemed unfair! It looked like chaos!

Then I noticed there were some things I really loved and some I hated, and most of the time I didn't know why. At that time, I loved everything Afro-American, Native American, Persian, and Tibetan, and hated everything German. I was also faintly repulsed by tall, blond men. I didn't think I was prejudiced, so why be repulsed by tall, blond men and Germans? Out of ten years living in Europe, I spent one night in Germany. That night I was so terrified that I barricaded my hotel room door with a dresser and chairs. Definitely not rational!

First with the help of friends guiding me, and then alone, I slowly began to remember experiences that we sometimes call past lives, personal archetypes, or parallel lives.

I remembered having been a German Jew who died at Buchenwald. After remembering, slowly I began to understand. I was judging Germans as they had judged me. They made Jews separate. I made Germans separate. There is a

"Hitler" in me—the part of me that judges. I forgave myself for making that separation and now appreciate Germans, and tall, blond men, as much as anyone else.

There is a "Hitler" in each of us. It's the part that keeps us separate from each other, from our kinship with all of life.

Perhaps the Jews and Germans were sacrificed to remind us of our common humanity—to give us another chance to remember to love. Will we listen to the gentle teaching of love, or will we create something horrible to remind us again? It's our choice. At each moment of our lives, you and I must choose between love and fear. If we don't choose love consciously, fear wins by default.

Gradually I began to experience life as a wave of energy, now creating in form, now dissolving into formlessness. The love, justice, freedom, peace, and joy we dream of are possible for everyone if we're moving toward realizing them over a number of lifetimes. I began to understand that what I'd interpreted as chaos were opportunities to learn.

I began to understand that all our concepts and beliefs about life, including my own, are not to be taken too seriously. They're helpful, if limited, frames of reference that give us a sense of purpose and direction. They point us toward experiencing everything as one. They aren't the experience. They too dissolve in the union with all that is. So, one set of beliefs is temporarily as useful as another as long as it makes the heart glad and leaves room for the beliefs of those who differ.

I know again in my heart that death is just a word we invented to describe leaving a body we no longer need. Life is endless...only the form changes.

And let us, above all things, never forget that in due course the dead will come back, and we never know when we shall see looking out at us from the eyes of a little child a soul we have know. Let us therefore...turn it to the endeavor of making the world a better place for the return of those we love.

—Dion Fortune
Through the Gates of Death

IF YOU WANT TO HELP

If *Coming Home* has helped your family to have a positive experience with caring for a dying loved at home, please consider passing on what you've learned to other people. Millions of people say they'd like to die at home, but most lack the information they need to do so. Here are some things you can do:

1. Recommend *Coming Home* to family members, friends, colleagues, hospices, women's groups, churches, synagogues, mosques, medical schools, cancer support groups, or other support groups.
2. Check if *Coming Home* is in your local library. If not, either donate a book, or suggest to the library that they add *Coming Home* to their collection. Ask your friends or family in other states to do this as well.
4. Encourage your local independent or chain bookstore to carry this book.
5. Write a book review for *Coming Home* for Amazon .com, Barnes & Noble, Borders, or a blog. Your candid comments will help.
6. Look for my new book, *Lighten Up: Seven Ways to Kick the Suffering Habit,* which will soon be available online and at your local bookstore.

Thank you,
Deborah

ACKNOWLEDGMENTS

Over the long life of this book, many people have contributed to it, from families caring for dying loved ones at home, to editors and publishers. The person who has been family, friend, and supporter of this book from its birth is Eve Muir. Her support has been a joy and made this new edition possible.

I am very grateful for Eugenia Chambers, RN, director of nursing at Community Hospice in New Orleans, for her invaluable help in updating the medical chapter to reflect the newest medical practices. Thank you to everyone at BookPros for your patience and skill in shepherding the publication of the fourth edition.

APPENDIX A
HOSPICE PHYSICIAN'S STANDING ORDERS SAMPLE FORM

Patient______________________________ Benefit period from ______________ to ______________

The orders as specified below will be followed unless otherwise noted. Dx:_____________________

Abrasions: Wash with antibacterial soap and water, apply Neosporin or Polysporin ointment BID x 7 days. Anxiety: Vistaril oral suspension 25mg/5 ml. 1–2 tsp qid PRN. Dispense 240cc. Refill x1. Or Ativan 0.5mg po q 4–6 hrs. #30. No refills.

Bladder: Use condom catheter or indwelling catheter to bedside drain for urinary incontinence. Discontinue condom catheter if penis irritation occurs. Catheterize patient with foley catheter size __/__ for inability to urinate. Change beside drainage bag every 2 weeks. Change catheter every month and PRN. Irrigate catheter with normal saline PRN or Acetic acid 25% if increased mucous production, sedimentation, or hematuria every day. Azo Standard 2 tabs TID x 2 days if patient complains of burning sensation after catheterization.

Constipation: Laxative of choice. Fleets Enema or SSE if no results from laxative. Rectal examination and manual removal of fecal impaction followed by Senokot tabs po BID.

Cough: Over-the-counter cough medicine of choice per package instructions. Contact MD for persistent cough.

Diarrhea: Kaopectate or Immodium AD as per directions on package.

DME: Nurse may order as needed.

Fever: Acetaminophen 650–1000mg po or rectally q 4 hrs. PNG fever>or = to 100.4 orally.

GI distress: Emetrol as per package directions for nausea. Persistent nausea and vomiting use Phenergan 25mg po or rectally 1 4–6 hrs. PRN. For indigestion or heartburn, antacid of choice per package directions. For unrelieved symptoms or vomiting, contact physician.

Hemorrhoids: Annusol suppository 1 hrs x 3 and Tuck pads.

Increased Secretions: Hyoscyamine 1 tab sublingual q 6 hrs. PRN.

Insomnia: Benadryl 25mg po qhs PRN.

Itching: Benadryl 25mg po q 4 hr. PRN. If itching last more than 2 days, notify MD.

Nasal Congestion: Saltwater nose drops QID x 2 days then if still with congestions, notify MD.

Oral Monilial Plaques: Nystatin oral suspension 5cc QID (swish and swallow) for oral candidiasis. Dispense 14-day supply. If initial infection severe or unsatisfactory response to above after 3 days, call MD.

Pain: Mild: Acetaminophen 650–1000mg q 4 hr. PRN or Ibuprofen 200–600mg q 6 hr. PRN. Moderate: Tylenol #3 1–2 tablets q 4 hr. po PRN. Dispense 40. No refills. If allergic to codeine, Darvocet N 100mg q 4 hrs. PRN po. Dispense 30. No refills. Severe: Notify MD.

Administer pain medication as ordered. If no relief in an hour repeat ½ original dosage and give 1 and ½ original dose thereafter.

Pressure Sores: Clean wound with normal saline, removing as much exudates as possible, pat dry, measure and stage wound. Apply DuoDERM and change every 5–7 days. For wounds with excessive drainage, notify MD.

Respiratory Distress: Oxygen at 2–3 LPM via NC PRN. If symptoms not relieved on stated liter flow, notify MD.

Skin Care: Keep skin clean and dry. Apply moisture barrier cream or patient's lotion of choice. Instruct on frequent position changes. Use APP as needed.
Skin Tears: Clean with normal saline removing as much exudates as possible, pat dry, apply Vigilon and Kerlex.
Sprains: Use cold packs PRN x 24 hrs. then warm packs PRN x 2 days. Notify MD if nurse suspects fracture, severe sprain, or if still painful in 2 days. Limit physical activity.
Sore Throat: Saltwater gargles QID x 3 days and Chloraseptic spray or lozenge QID x 3 days then if still symptomatic or patient running fever, notify MD.
Yeast Infections: Monostat cream per package directions.

EMERGENCY ADMIT PACK may be placed in patient home and initiated by the nurse as needed containing the following medications:

Acetaminophen Suppositories 650mg #2 1 every 4–6 hrs. PRN.

Prochlorperazine Suppositories 25mg #2 1 every 4–6 hrs. and PRN.

Hyoscyamine 0.125mg SL tabs. #9 1 every 6 hrs. PRN.

Lorazepan Intensol 2mg/ml 10cc ½ to 1cc po every 4–6 hrs. PRN.

Morphine Concentrate 20mg/ml 10cc ½ to 1cc po every 2–4 hrs. PRN.

Temazepan 15mg #4 1 po qhs PRN.

Senna 8.6/50mg #12 1–2 po as directed. ______________
______________ date________
Verbal Order by:______________________________
date________
Attending Physician______________________________
date________

APPENDIX B
SAMPLE ADVANCE DIRECTIVE

DIRECTIVE TO PHYSICIANS

Directive made this ______the day of _____ in the year _____.
I,__________________, being of sound mind, willfully and voluntarily make known my desire that my life shall not be artificially prolonged under the circumstances set forth in this directive.

1. If at any time I should have an incurable or irreversible condition caused by injury, disease, or illness certified to be a terminal condition by two physicians, and if the application of life-sustaining procedures would serve only to artificially postpone the moment of my death, and if my attending physician determines that my death is imminent or will result within a relatively short time without the application of life-sustaining procedures, I ask that those procedures be withheld or withdrawn, and that I be permitted to die naturally.
2. In the absence of my ability to give directions regarding the use of those life-sustaining procedures, it is my intention that this directive be honored by my family and physicians as the final expression of my legal right to refuse medical or surgical treatment and accept the consequences from that refusal.
3. I understand the full import of this directive and I am emotionally and mentally competent to make this directive.

4. I understand that I may revoke this directive at any time.
5. I request that only comfort care be provided to me, no antibiotics, no artificial nutrition, no mechanical ventilation, and no hydration. It is my strong preference to be allowed to die outside of a care facility if possible, even if that preference is determined by my physician to shorten my period of dying. The only condition under which I desire these preferences for end-of-life care to be altered is in the case of possible organ and tissue donation. I request that any and all organs and tissue that may be salvaged be provided for transplant. My remains may then be cremated.

Signed ______________________________ in the City of ____________ Date_______________

I am not a person designated by the declarant to make a treatment decision. I am not related to the declarant by blood or marriage. I would not be entitled to any portion of the declarant's estate on the declarant's death. I am not the attending physician of the declarant or an employee of the attending physician. I have no claim against any portion of the declarant's estate on the declarant's death. Furthermore, if I am an employee of the health care facility in which the declarant is a patient, I am not involved in providing direct patient care to the declarant and am not an officer, director, partner, or business office employee of the heath care facility or of any parent organization of the health care facility.

Witness____

Witness____.

APPENDIX C
USEFUL RESOURCES

American Association of Retired People (AARP). www.aarp.org.

AARP provides a wealth of information on useful subjects from caregiving to the latest changes to Medicare. Phone: (888) 687-2277.

Association for Death Education and Counseling (ADEC). www.adec.org.

This professional organization dedicated to death education, bereavement counseling, and care of the dying has excellent information on bereavement rituals. Phone: (847) 509-0403.

Family Caregiver Alliance (FCA). www.caregiver.org.

A national organization that provides advice, strategies, and services for helping caregivers. Web site includes navigator to connect you to caregiver services in your state. Phone: (800) 445-8106.

CaringBridge. www.Caringbridge.org.

On this site you can quickly and easily set up a free, private, personalized web site to help you share up-to-date information on the dying process you are living with family and friends. Phone: (651) 452-7940.

Caring Connections. www.caringinfo@nhpco.org.

Part of the National Hospice and Palliative Care Organization, this group provides free advance directives with instructions; information on caring for the dying and grieving a loss; and has a hospice locator link. Phone: (800) 658-8898.

Compassionate Friends, The (TCF). www.compassionatefriends.org

Their mission is to assist families—parents, grandparents, and siblings—who are grieving the death of a child. Phone: (877) 969-0010 to locate a local chapter.

Eldercare Locator. www.eldercare.gov.

A service of the U.S. Administration on Aging, the locator links you to community-based organizations near you that focus on end-of-life care. Phone: (800) 677-1116.

Funeral Consumers' Alliance (FCA). www.funerals.org.

This nonprofit grassroots organization protects consumers' right to choose affordable, meaningful, and dignified funerals and has a locator to connect you with a local group. Phone: (800) 765-0107.

Green Burial Council (GBC). www.greenburialcouncil.org.

The GBC is working toward making burial more sustainable, economically viable, and meaningful. A locator connects you to approved funeral providers, cemeteries, cremation services, and products. Phone: (888) 966-3330.

Legal Zoom. www.legalzoom.com.

This helpful site was founded by attorneys to provide reasonably priced legal services. Phone: (800) 773-0888.

Hospice Foundation of America (HFA).
www.hospicefoundation.org.

HFA promotes hospice care, educates professionals, and provides useful information to help family with end-of-life information. Phone: (800) 854-3402.

National Hospice and Palliative Care Organization (NHPCO).
www.nhpco.org.

NHPCO provides information about end-of-life issues and state-specific advance directives. Phone: (800) 658-8898.

APPENDIX D
WRITING YOUR CHILD'S STORY

This suggestion written by Margaret Gerner, a parent of a child who died, appeared in a 1994 *Compassionate Friends* newsletter, St. Louis, Missouri.

"The possibility of forgetting even the smallest detail of our child's life is a fear most of us have. In truth, over the months and years many of these details do dim. Writing them down is a way to keep from losing these memories. This way we will not only have a permanent remembrance of our child for ourselves, but this will be a legacy for the other brothers and sisters. Here are some suggestions.

- Write in a spiral notebook.
- Begin at the beginning. Write all the details of your child's life from birth through the death day.
- Use your child's pictures to help remind you of occasions and happenings over the years. Ask friends and relatives to tell you anything they remember about your child. Also write any thoughts and feelings you remember having at the time.
- Record the 'bad' things your child said and did in his/her life, as well as the 'good' things so you can remember him/her as a real person.
- Write about your child's death. Record as many details surrounding it as you care to retell. Write about the days before the burial, the funeral, the days after, two weeks, a month, and so on. Record how others helped.
- Write a letter to your child, and include:

What I wish I had said to you.
What I wish I had done.
What I wish you would have done.
What I wish I could ask you.
What I wish I hadn't said to you.
What I wish I had not done.
What I wish you had not done.
What I would like to tell you.

- Pour out your feelings to your child. Tell him/her of your anger, your guilts. Tell your child how you love her/him. Tell your child GOODBYE.

Don't worry about whether you write well or not. Don't worry about form or grammar. Just write.

Keep your notebook handy. Write any time you want to say something to him/her, or when you remember some detail. The times you have trouble sleeping write down the things that keep coming into your mind. Writing about your child or to your child will be emotional. It will probably make you cry. Don't let this stop you. Crying will help you with your grief work.

Remember, 'writing is just talking written down.'"

BIBLIOGRAPHY

About Dying. A Scriptographic Booklet. New Haven, CT: Channing L. Bete Co., 1978.

Ars Moriendi (Dying Arts). Walter J. Johnson edition. (One of the world's first do-it-yourself books, it taught the art of dying. It was originally published in Florence in 1488. A modern English edition was published by Arno Press, New York, 1977.)

Blake, William. *Notebook.* Edited by Geoffrey Keynes. Totowa, NJ: Cooper Square Publishing, 1971.

Boone, J. Allen. *Kinship with All Life.* New York: Harper and Row, 1976.

Bricklin, Mark. *The Practical Encyclopedia of Natural Healing.* Rodale Press: Emmaus, PA.

Caxton, William (translator). *Art and Craft to Knewe Ye Well to Dye.* Westminster, England, 1490. (This book includes instructions for everything from the art of blowing your nose to weeping well.)

Coughlin, George G. *Law for the Layman.* New York: Harper and Row, 1975.

Cousin, Norman. *Anatomy of an Illness as Perceived by the Patient: Reflections on Healing and Regeneration.* New York: W.W. Norton and Co., 1979.

Fortune, Dion. *Through the Gates of Death.* York Beach, ME: Samuel Weiser, 1968.

Frankl, Viktor E. *Man's Search for Meaning: An Introduction to Logotherapy.* Boston, MA: Beacon Press, 1959. (Victor Frankl was a psychiatrist who survived Auschwitz and Dachau. After his experiences there, he stated, "The salvation of man is through love and in love.")

Fynn. *Mister God, This Is Anna.* New York: Ballantine Books, 1974.

Gibran, Kahlil. *The Prophet.* New York: Alfred A. Knopf, 1967.

The Gospel According to Thomas. New York: Harper and Row, 1957.

Gray, V. Ruth. *Dealing with Death and Dying, Some Psychosocial Needs.* Jenkintown, PA: Nursing 77 Books, Nursing Skill Book Service, 1978.

Grof, Stanislav and Joan Halifax. *The Human Encounter with Death.* New York: E.P. Dutton, 1978.

Heline, Corinne. "Color and Music in the New Age." *New Age Magazine,* 1964.

Holland, Canon Scott. *Facts of the Faith.*

Huxley, Laura. *This Timeless Moment.* Millbrae, CA: Celestial Arts, 1975.

Illich, Ivan. *Medical Nemesis: The Expropriation of Health.* New York: Pantheon, 1976.

Internal Revenue Service. *A Guide to Federal Estate and Gift Taxation* (#448), *Tax Information to Survivors* (#559).

Jampolsky, Gerald. *Love Is Letting Go of Fear.* Millbrae, CA: Celestial Arts, 1979.

Khan, Hazrat Inayat. *The Purpose of Life.* San Francisco, CA: The Rainbow Bridge Bookstore, 1973.

Lack, Sylvia A. *Psychosocial Care of the Dying Patient.* New York: McGraw Hill, 1978. (Originally a paper given before the First National Training Conference for Physicians on Psychosocial Care of the Dying Patient, April 29, 1976.)

LeShan, Eda. *Learning to Say Goodbye.* New York: Macmillan, 1976.

Levine, Stephen. *The Gradual Awakening.* New York: Doubleday, 1979.

Lipnack, Jessica. "Dying: New Age Readers Respond." *New Age Magazine,* March, 1978.

Lopez, Barry (editor). "The American Indian Mind." *Omni Magazine,* Sept–Oct, 1978.

Maclean, Dorothy. *To Hear the Angels Sing.* Findhorn Publications, 1980.

Marback, Ethel. *The Cabbage Moth and the Shamrock.* La Jolla, CA: Star and Elephant Books, Green Tiger Press, 1978.

Miriam, Satya. *Healing is Transformation: The Opening of the Rose.* New York: Baraka Books, 1978.

Moody, Raymond, MD. *Life After Life.* Harrisburg, PA: Stackpole Books, 1976.

Morgan, Ernest. *A Manual of Death Education and Simple Burial.* Burnsville, NC: Celo Press, 1977.

Muggeridge, Malcolm. *Something Beautiful for God.* New York: Doubleday, 1977.

Muir, John. *The Velvet Monkey Wrench.* Santa Fe, NM: John Muir Publications, 1973.

Neihard, John G. *Black Elk Speaks.* Lincoln, NB: University of Nebraska Press, 1961.

Osis, Dr. Karlis and Erlendur Haraldsson. "Deathbed Observations by Physicians and Nurse: A Cross-Cultural Survey." *The Journal for the American Society of Psychical Research,* 1961.

Perry, Whittall N. *A Treasury of Traditional Wisdom.* New York: Simon and Schuster, 1972.

"Here Comes a Fresh Breeze of God," *Rajneesh Foundation Newsletter,* Volume III, #18, Sept. 16, 1977.

Seiver, George. *The Man and His Mind.* New York: Harper and Row, 1976.

Stern, Phillip. *Lawyers on Trial.* New York: Time Books, 1980.

Sultanoff, Barry. "Reflections." *The Movement Newspaper,* May, 1986.

NOTES

Preface

1. *NHPCO Facts and Figures: Hospice Care in America* (Alexandria, VA: National Hospice and Palliative Care Organization, October 2009), 3.
2. Quoted in *NHPCO Facts and Figures* (October 2009), 5.
3. American Association of Retired Persons, *AARP Bulletin,* June 2008, 3.

Chapter 1

1. Lynette Grouse, "Improving quality of life by managing cancer pain," National Cancer Institute, 2005, http://www.cancer.gov.
2. This poem has been attributed at different times to J.T. Wiggins (an English emigrant to America); two Americans, Mary E. Fry and Marianne Reinhardt; and more recently to Stephen Cummins, a British soldier killed in Northern Ireland who left a copy for his relatives. Others claim it is a Navajo burial prayer.

Chapter 3

1. Cousins was editor of *The Saturday Review* and author of *Anatomy of Illness,* a biographical book about how he healed himself of a life-threatening disease using humor.

2. Ivan Illich, *Medical Nemesis: The Expropriation of Health* (New York: Pantheon Books, 1976).
3. "A Symposium: The Quinlan Case, 10 Years Later; When Sophisticated Medicine Does More Harm than Good," *New York Times,* March 30, 1986.
4. *NHPCO Facts and Figures: Hospice Care in America* (Alexandria, VA: National Hospice and Palliative Care Organization, October 2009), 8.
5. "Opinion 2.20—Withholding or Withdrawing Life-Sustaining Medical Treatment," American Medical Association, http://www.ama-assn.org/ama/pub/physician-resources/medical-ethics/code-medical-ethics/opinion220.shtml.
6. *NHPCO Facts and Figures* (October 2009), 4.
7. *NHPCO Facts and Figures* (October 2009).
8. Malcolm Muggeridge, *Something Beautiful for God* (New York: Harper & Row, 1971), 99.

Chapter 4

1. Department of Veterans Affairs, http://www.vba.va.gov/bln/21/Rates/pen0101.htm.

Chapter 5

1. U.S. Census Bureau, "The 2010 Statistical Abstract," http://www.census.gov/compendia/statab/2010/tables/10s0078.pdf.

Chapter 6

1. Merry N. Miller, MD, "The painful truth: physicians are not invincible," *Southern Medical Journal* (2000), 1.

2. Lynette Grouse, "Improving quality of life by managing cancer pain," National Cancer Institute, 2005, www.cancer.gov.

3. P. Whitcar, MD, "Managing pain in the dying patient," The Academy of American Physicians, 2000, www.aafp.

4. Ivan Illich, *Medical Nemesis: The Expropriation of Health* (New York: Pantheon Books, 1976), 140.

5. Stanislav Grof and Joan Halifax, *The Human Encounter with Death* (New York: E. P. Dutton, 1978).

Chapter 7

1. Sylvia Lack, MD, "The psychosocial care of the dying patient," First National Training Conference for Physicians on Psychosocial Care of the Dying Patient, 1976.

2. "This Bill of Rights was created at a workshop on the terminally ill patient and the helping person in Lansing, Michigan, sponsored by the Southwestern Michigan Inservice Education Council and conducted by Amelia J. Barbus, associate professor of nursing, Wayne State University, in 1975." Quoted in Betty Ferrell, "An Overview of Palliative Nursing Care," *American Journal of Nursing,* http://journals.lww.com/ajnonline/Fulltext/2002/05000/An_Overview_of_Palliative_Nursing_Care__Studies.30.aspx.

Chapter 8

1. Barry Lopez, ed., "The American Indian Mind," *Omni Magazine,* Sept–Oct, 1978.

Chapter 10

1. Kübler-Ross, *On Death and Dying* (New York: Scribner, 2003), 149.

Chapter 11

1. "Introduction to Estate and Gift Taxes," IRS Publication 950, December 2009, http://www.irs.gov/pub/irs-pdf/p950.pdf.

Chapter 12

1. Marvin Meyer, *The Gospel of Thomas* (San Francisco: Harper Collins Publishers, 1992), 35.

Chapter 14

1. "Statistics," National Funeral Directors Association, http://www.nfda.org/media-center/statisticsreports.html#cfacts.
2. "2006 NFDA General Price List Survey" (June 2008), quoted on "Statistics," National Funeral Directors Association, http://www.nfda.org/about-funeral-service/trends-and-statistics.html.

Chapter 15

1. David W. Moore, "Three in Four Americans Believe in Paranormal," Gallup, June 16, 2005, http://www.gallup.com/poll/16915/three-four-americans-believe-paranormal.aspx.

Chapter 16

1. Bill Newcott, "Life after death," *AARP The Magazine*, Sept/Oct, 2007.
2. "The Genographic Project," National Geographic Society, https://genographic.nationalgeographic.com/genographic/

lan/en/index.html.

3. The edict of the Second Council of Constantinople said, "Whosoever shall support the mythical doctrine of the preexistence of the soul and the consequent wonderful opinion of its return, let him be anathema."
4. Pope Virgilius never authorized the "anathema" but it was generally believed that he had. Because the Church never made an "official" statement against reincarnation, perhaps it's possible for practicing Catholics to believe in reincarnation without being in technical disagreement with Church doctrine.
5. "Grief During Childhood," American Cancer Society, http://ww3.cancer.org/docroot/MBC/content/MBC_4_1X_Grief_During_Childhood.asp?sitearea=MBC.

NOTES

NOTES

NOTES

NOTES

NOTES

NOTES

NOTES

NOTES

NOTES

NOTES

NOTES